"In our rapidly evolving new age of marijuana appreciation and education, *How to Smoke Pot (Properly)* provides a thoughtful, historical, and comprehensive account of all things cannabis. Filled with useful information that encompasses just about every situation imaginable, from rolling your first joint to properly passing one in a foreign land with new friends, David Bienenstock expresses his passion and commitment in a way only someone dedicated to keeping it weird possibly can."

— Alex Lifeson, guitarist of Rush

"*How to Smoke Pot (Properly)* is a delightful book proclaiming that marijuana smoking can be an exhilarating, creative experience. David Bienenstock sets the tone in his introduction when he says, 'It's no longer sufficient to talk about the harms of marijuana prohibition. We've got to start loudly and proudly celebrating the many serious benefits this plant brings into our lives and communities.'"

— Keith Stroup, NORML founder and legal counsel

"It's a healthy development that society has reached the point where it needed this book, and I'm glad someone of David Bienenstock's eloquence and experience has written it."

— Doug Fine, author of *Farewell, My Subaru*; *Too High to Fail*; and *Hemp Bound*

"Covering history, etiquette, medicine, consumption, and safety, this is a complete examination of cannabis today, penned by a master of prose. . . . I love this book!"

— Jorge Cervantes, bestselling author of *Marijuana Horticulture*

HOW TO SMOKE POT (PROPERLY)

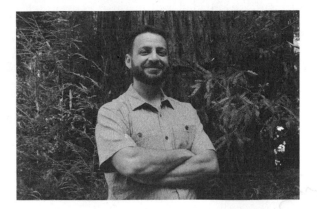

DAVID BIENENSTOCK is the former West Coast editor of *High Times* magazine and has more recently grown a following as a journalist and video host/producer at VICE, where he writes the Weed Eater column and produces a video series called *Bong Appetit*. He's appeared as a cannabis expert on NPR, Fox News, MSNBC, CNN, CNBC, and HBO and has been quoted in *Salon, GQ, Fast Company, Adweek, Playboy,* and *The Nation.* For more information, visit www.davidbienenstock.com, or follow him on Twitter at @pot_handbook.

Praise for
How to Smoke Pot Properly

"It's refreshing, in the midst of our binge culture, to find a voice that clearly articulates the benefits and pitfalls of cannabis enthusiasm while strongly encouraging responsible consumption and cultivation. There is no better spokesperson for the cannabis-positive lifestyle in the post-prohibition era than David Bienenstock."
—Ben Sinclair, cocreator and star of the HBO original series *High Maintenance*

HOW TO
SMOKE POT

(Properly)

A HIGHBROW GUIDE TO GETTING HIGH

DAVID BIENENSTOCK

A PLUME BOOK

PLUME

An imprint of Penguin Random House LLC
375 Hudson Street
New York, New York 10014

Credit for photo on p. 212 © 1971, 2015 by George Shelton.
First published 1971 as back cover of *The Collected Adventures of the Fabulous
Furry Freak Brothers* by Rip Off Press, San Francisco, California.

P REGISTERED TRADEMARK — MARCA REGISTRADA

LIBRARY OF CONGRESS CATALOGING-IN-PUBLICATION DATA
Bienenstock, David, author.
How to smoke pot (properly) : a highbrow guide to
getting high / David Bienenstock.
pages cm
Includes bibliographical references.
ISBN 978-0-14-751708-1
1. Marijuana.   2. Marijuana abuse.   3. Drug paraphernalia.   I. Title.
HV5822.M3B457   2016
394.1'4 — dc23
2015033906

Printed in the United States of America
1   3   5   7   9   10   8   6   4   2

Illustrations by Samantha Russo

Book design by Sabrina Bowers

To Elise, my partner in every step of this journey.
And to Dr. Lester Grinspoon,
for helping the world reconsider marijuana.

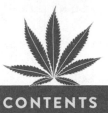

CONTENTS

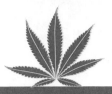

AUTHOR'S NOTE

While this is a wholly new work, the author acknowledges that in certain places it briefly recounts adventures and interviews undertaken while working as an on-staff editor at *High Times* or as a freelance reporter and video host/producer with VICE media. In each instance, this fact is made directly transparent to the reader in the main text.

There are also a small number of instances where a short passage of the author's own writing has been retained whole or mostly whole from one of these earlier works. This has been done with all necessary permission from the original publisher and represents a small percentage of the overall text.

The author wishes to thank both *High Times* and VICE for their dedication to quality marijuana journalism and for their years of support and encouragement.

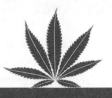

*It would be wryly interesting, if in
human history the cultivation of
marijuana led generally to the
invention of agriculture, and thereby
to civilization.*
   —CARL SAGAN, *DRAGONS OF EDEN*

WINNING THE PEACE

Once literally demonized as "the devil's lettuce," and linked
to all manner of deviant behavior by the establishment's shame-
less anti-pot propaganda campaigns, *Cannabis sativa* has lately
been enjoying a long-overdue Renaissance. Most Americans
now live in a state with some type of medical-marijuana law in
place, while outright legalization—which has already taken root
in Colorado, Washington, Alaska, Oregon, and Washington,
DC—appears set to spread like a grassfire.

Still, too many otherwise law-abiding adults continue to face
persecution for the simple love of a plant. And after more than
a decade spent reporting on marijuana every day, I know all too
well that as long as any one of us is oppressed, none truly blaze
free. But as society's perception of marijuana rapidly evolves,
the world's long-suffering herbal enthusiasts can at last look
forward to a time when nobody faces harsh punishment for

consuming, growing, sharing, or even selling this most won-
drous weed. A glorious day when cannabis is duly recognized
as a lifesaving medicine, an incredibly nutritious food, an amazingly useful industrial crop, a far safer alternative to alcohol, a
renewable energy source, and an all-around enhancer of life's
pleasures.

Keep in mind, for roughly 10,000 years, humanity revered the
herb for these and many other reasons. Only relatively recently
has cannabis become the target of a coordinated global eradication campaign. No inherent property of the species can explain
this dramatic reversal, until you realize that the War on Weed
stems not from an attempt to lessen marijuana's harms, but rather
to suppress its benefits—an insidious plot to protect the pharmaceutical industry, Big Tobacco, the booze barons, and the plastic
industrial complex from unwanted competition while building
up a modern police state right under our noses. And they would
have gotten away with it too, if it wasn't for us meddlesome
stoners. For together, we've engaged in a highly effective civil-
disobedience campaign to end this senseless and self-destructive
prohibition against an incredibly beneficial botanical.

From the growers, smugglers, and dealers who risk their
freedom making sure marijuana survives the government's pot
pogrom, to the activists who stand up for our right to be treated
like customers instead of criminals, to the many brave patients
who step forward to tell the world how marijuana helps them
heal, to those who simply roll a joint in defiance of the law, the
seeds of this reefer revolution have been scattered far and wide,
and now a joyous harvest draws near.

We've officially reached the beginning of the end of pot prohibition. At which point the key question becomes: *What's
next?* Will cannabis become just another corporatized commod-
ity, controlled by Philip Morris and Monsanto? Or will the
weed heads band together to keep out the greed heads?

And what will become of the weed heads themselves? Will cannabis consumers remain second-class citizens, or will our vibrant, innovative, life-affirming underground culture at last fully emerge from the shadows and take its rightful place at the head of the table?

A lot depends on how the world views not just marijuana but those who choose to consume it. We're the ones who've been right about weed all along, of course, but the corrupt powers that be don't want to admit that they've been wrong. Because then someone might hold them accountable for all the millions of people arrested and put in prison for a big lie; all the cancer patients who needlessly suffered through chemo when a few puffs could have helped immensely; all the no-knock raids, lying narcs, sleazy informants, warrantless surveillance, racial profiling, ruined lives, and wasted resources.

So now the media's trying to sell us a new story, about how Big Business and government regulators are working together to "legitimize" marijuana. And we sure as hell can't let them get away with *that*. Not after all we've suffered and sacrificed. Which means it's high time we start to redefine this debate. It's no longer sufficient to talk about the harms of marijuana prohibition. We've got to start loudly and proudly celebrating the many serious benefits this plant brings into our lives and communities.

"The stone that the builder refuse, will always be the head cornerstone," Bob Marley once sang, echoing the words of Psalm 118:22. And while it's unclear if he was specifically referring to ganja, he might as well have been. Because this most maligned and misconstrued herb not only isn't *bad*, it may in fact be our last best chance to heal the planet and fix our fucked-up society before it's too late.

So whether you've been smoking tea longer than Willie Nelson or just took your first puff last week, my hope is that by the end of this book, you'll learn to see cannabis not just as a plea-sure and a political cause, but also as the "cornerstone" of a new and better way of life.

Hey, it worked for me.

MEET YOUR GANJA GUIDE

As an editor at *High Times* magazine for ten years, and more recently as a weed columnist and frequent contributor at VICE, I've had the great privilege of interviewing an amazing array of high-functioning marijuana thought leaders from all walks of life, many of whom you'll get to meet in these pages. And I can con-fidently affirm that in addition to a deep respect for the cannabis plant, these growers, doctors, dealers, healers, smugglers, scien-tists, celebrities, entrepreneurs, patients, prisoners, politicians, artists, and philosophers all share a highly enlightened approach to existence—one that allows them to stay true to themselves in a world that's both corrupt and corrupting.

Not that everybody must get stoned to achieve this exalted plane of being, or that getting high *necessarily* renders such gifts, but I do believe smoking pot *properly* can help most people learn to live a more authentic, rewarding life. At least, that's been my experience. I first tried marijuana as an angry young man who saw a lot of injustice in the world, and not much hope for fixing it. I had trouble fitting in, and wasn't sure I wanted to. I'd had plenty to drink by that point, and found alcohol typi-cally made matters worse (though feel free to buy me a beer now).

Aside from a lot of laughing, I don't recall anything out of the ordinary happening the night I surrendered my herbal vir-ginity. A few friends and I passed around a pipe made from a cored-out apple and shot the shit in the woods behind a bowl-ing alley—a fairly typical Friday night for me, then and now. Except that everything we said turned out to be off-the-charts hilarious, and perhaps not just in our own stoned minds.

After all, renowned French poet Charles Baudelaire noted a similar phenomenon at the regular meetings of Paris's famed Club des Hashischins (hashish-eaters club), which gathered fre-quently in the mid-1800s to drink a special blend of strong cof-fee, hashish, nutmeg, cloves, cinnamon, pistachio, orange juice, cantharides, sugar, and butter. Luminary members included Al-exandre Dumas, Victor Hugo, and Honoré de Balzac, though from Baudelaire's description, even the lesser lights among them somehow managed to keep up with the club's marijuana-infused milieu of witty repartee.

"It sometimes happens that people completely unsuited for word-play will improvise an endless string of puns and wholly improbable idea relationships fit to outdo the ablest masters of this preposterous craft," Baudelaire wrote in *Artificial Paradises* of his experiences as a hashish-laced coffee drinker. "But after a few minutes, the relation between ideas becomes so vague, and the thread of thoughts grows so tenuous, that only your cohorts . . . can understand you."

What I remember best from my own first time getting high, however, wasn't all that amazing wisecracking we managed to pull off but rather the point where I started laughing so hard that I couldn't remember what, exactly, I was laughing at. Which only made me laugh harder, until it grew into some kind of cos-mic guffaw. And then I realized I was laughing at myself—maybe for the first time in my life—and it felt really good. Even the next day, no longer high, I felt cleansed. All the same things still made me just as angry, but I could somehow deal with them—and myself—a lot better. As Bob Marley once said in an interview, "When you smoke the herb, it reveals you to yourself."

And Jah only knows where I'd be now and what I'd be doing with my life without that experience and the many stoned epiphanies that followed. I've actually thought a lot about where a potless parallel universe might have taken me, but I'm not sure I'd ever really want to go there. I certainly wouldn't trade this life for any other. After all, I get to spend every day (and too many nights) writing about the most amazing life-form in the known universe. And now I get to share all I've learned and experienced along the way with you. And hopefully set you off on your own marijuana adventure, or help you make the most of the one you're already having.

UTILIZE IT!

I once asked Grammy-winning reggae artist (and son of Bob) Damian Marley if marijuana is part of his creative process. He quickly replied: "Ganja is part of my every process."

Which doesn't mean he smokes herb all day, every day (although he *was* puffing on a rather sizable spliff at the time). It means cannabis has positively, permanently affected the way he sees the world, whether he's high or not. And really, when we talk about smoking pot *properly*, more than anything else, that's what's required. You must learn to *utilize* your high, even when you're not high.

"The illegality of cannabis," famed astronomer Carl Sagan once observed, in a 1969 essay, "is an outrageous impediment to full utilization of a drug which helps produce the serenity and insight, sensitivity and fellowship so desperately needed in this increasingly mad and dangerous world."

Marijuana legalization, therefore, it stands to reason, makes the world a little less mad and dangerous with each new territory that's liberated from this terrible oppression. And make no mistake, that's exactly what we've suffered and continue to suffer—*oppression*. What else do you call it when armed representatives of the state kick down your door, shoot your dog, seize your children, deny you lifesaving medicine, and lock you in a cage, *over a plant*? All of which still happens with shocking regularity, and not in some distant realm run by a crazed despot, but in Kansas, which shares a more-than-two-hundred-mile-long border with the free state of Colorado.

The idea for this book, not coincidentally, was born in Denver, on January 1, 2014—the day America's first retail marijuana stores opened to anyone twenty-one and over, no matter where you live, and without a note from your doctor. Waiting in line that morning, in the snow, at dawn, as dozens of satellite-equipped TV trucks sat idling in front of 3D Cannabis Center, I knew the whole world was about to change irrevocably the instant all those images of peaceful people waiting patiently to buy legal weed were beamed out into the universe.

Reporter's notebook in hand, working on a VICE story called "I Just Bought Legal Weed," I asked literally every single prospective cannabis consumer I met that day why they came to Colorado, including more than a few from Kansas, and nobody said "to buy pot." They all came to make history.

So it's not marijuana that's changing but society's understanding of marijuana. And those of us who were cannabis before it was cool must adapt or die too. Huge moneyed interests have already moved in and started taking over the growing and selling of the plant, and now they're setting their sights on our culture too. Backed by hedge-fund d-bags and spurred on by the media's endless breathless special reports on the legal pot "green rush," the Don Drapers of the world have schemed up a plan to transform sweet Mary Jane into yet another branding opportunity.

But it doesn't have to go down that way. Not if we all work together to preserve the egalitarian, freewheeling, antiestablishment roots of authentic underground marijuana culture while simultaneously growing up boldly into the light of true freedom. We can remain outlaws in spirit, with the added bonus of not having to actually break the law. We can even, at long last, seize the moral high ground from those who've made a tidy profit oppressing us. Because really, who would you trust to give you a square deal in this day and age: a Wall Street wheeler-dealer or your friendly neighborhood weed dealer?

And so, please think of this humble tome in your hands not just as a handbook or a guidebook but also as a call to (metaphorical) arms. Ours is a way of life worth defending and preserving. Which starts with knowing where we're at, and how we got here.

They say history is written by the victors, but most of the marijuana books I've seen come out since legalization became the new *L* word were penned by people who didn't give a damn about cannabis until they saw a market niche open up. Without exception, these works focus on the "high profits" to be made in legal pot, which very naturally seems like the big story to a bunch of Johnny-come-lately weed writers, because the modern pot biz is full of newbies and pretenders just like them.

But I think the *big* story is something much deeper. And it starts with asking two simple questions: *What has gone wrong in a society that wages a costly, dehumanizing, self-destructive war on a beneficial plant? And what might that same society have to gain by embracing cannabis instead of criminalizing it?*

To find out, together, we'll delve into the botany and chemistry of marijuana, discover the way the herb's bred, grown, harvested, and processed around the world, and learn how, exactly, marijuana heals the body, protects the mind, improves creativity, catalyzes epiphanies, and accesses higher consciousness. We'll also follow the natural life cycle of the species from farm to pipe; explore cannabis customs, culture, and travel; and discover how to best utilize and appreciate this truly blessed herb.

Plus, I've compiled dozens of "pro tips" from cannabis celebrities and herbal legends of the marijuana movement, who'll answer burning questions like *How can I land a legal pot job? Should I eat a THC-infused cookie before boarding the plane?* and *What's the best technique for rolling a joint in a windstorm?*

So what are you waiting for?

Oh yeah, of course, by all means go roll something up and get ready for a quick *high*-story lesson. (And if you don't know how to roll, most definitely skip to page 60 and then double back.)

ILLUSTRATED TIMELINE OF MARIJUANA HISTORY

Perhaps the world's oldest cultivated crop, *Cannabis sativa* has been planted, tended, and harvested for more than 10,000 years. According to researcher Martin A. Lee's authoritative *Smoke Signals: A Social History of Marijuana*, "ancient peoples during the Neolithic period found uses for virtually every part of the plant. . . . The stems and stalks provided fiber for cordage and cloth; the seeds, a key source of essential fatty acids and protein, were eaten as foods; and the roots, leaves and flowers were utilized in medicinal and ritual preparations."

Lee largely credits the weed-loving, widely migratory ancient Scythians with taking a species native to central Asia and spreading it across Eurasia and into Europe, citing a passage in

Herodotus's *Histories* (BCE 500) that describes Scythians of this far-gone era "howling with pleasure" in a hemp vapor bath. Which sounds like a pretty kickass way to hotbox a sweat lodge, if you ask me.

In time, the herb found a home in virtually every inhabited place on Earth, forever changing the course of world events in the process. So let's take a closer look at the hidden weed history your teachers never told you about.

BCE 6000

Earliest archeological evidence of cannabis used as a food source.

BCE 4000

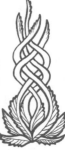

A well-preserved discovery in China's Zhejiang Province provides the earliest evidence of hemp's use in making textiles, though the practice may have originated far earlier.

BCE 2727

A revered figure to this day in China, where he's seen as the father of both modern agriculture and herbal medicine, Emperor Shennong makes the first recorded mention of medical marijuana while preparing one of the world's earliest pharmacopeias.

According to legend, Shennong—also known as "the divine farmer"—personally ingested hundreds of wild herbs in search of those with healing properties. *The Divine Farmer's Herb-Root Classic*, which compiled his findings, lists cannabis among the "supreme elixirs of immortality," praising its female flowers specifically as a superior treatment for "constipation, 'female weakness,' gout, malaria, rheumatism, and absentmindedness."

BCE 1200

The Atharvaveda, one of the four *Vedas* comprising the oldest scriptural Hindu text, provides the first known documentation of cannabis as a spiritual aid. Particularly associated with the playful god Shiva, cannabis is praised for bringing joy and relieving anxiety. Shiva is said to have discovered the restorative powers of the herb after falling asleep in the shade of a towering pot plant one hot afternoon, and then sampling its leaves upon waking.

BCE 500

A 2,500-year-old gravesite in Kazakhstan houses the remains of a couple who chose to be interred together along with their communal stash—a sacramental leather pouch full of wild pot seeds—presumably to ensure they'd still have weed to share in the afterlife.

BCE 300–100

Hemp spreads throughout Europe, where it's utilized both as a food source and to make textiles. By the fifteenth century, hemp rope and sails would give rise to the "Age of Discovery," when far-flung European explorers began "discovering," and subsequently violently subjugating, much of the rest of the world. (Might history have turned out differently if those colonialist Europeans had been smoking cannabis in addition to weaving it?)

900–1000

Cannabis spreads rapidly throughout the Middle East and Arabia in the form of concentrated hashish, spurring leading Islamic scholars of the day to debate whether it should be banned (alongside alcohol) on religious grounds, even though the Koran enforces no such direct prohibition.

1200

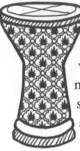

Arab traders introduce cannabis to the African continent for the first time. Called *dagga*, the herb was added in copious amounts to bonfires by Pygmies, Zulus, Hottentots, and other tribes, fueling some of the most epic drum circles and chanting sessions in history.

1253

Egyptian authorities initiate one of the first drug wars in history after a group of hashish-smoking Sufis set up shop in the middle of Cairo and plant a communal, municipal cannabis garden in a public park. Those caught growing weed faced capital punishment, while mere hashish eaters only had their teeth yanked out.

1378

Soudoun Scheikhouni, the emir of the Ottoman Empire and a brutal ruler, claims the consumption of cannabis leads to sloth, irreverence, and immorality, and issues one of the world's first edicts against the eating of hashish, thus earning the nickname "Emir Buzzkill."

1619

The Virginia Assembly (earliest predecessor to the US state of Virginia) passes a law requiring every productive farm within its jurisdiction to plant and harvest hemp, a crop that's also accepted as legal tender. Hemp would become a key factor in the rise of the colonies as an economic power, and then play a huge role in making the American War of Independence possible by supplying the revolutionaries with a homegrown source of rope, sails, and other vital military resources, plus food, medicine, and textiles, with enough of the crop left over to trade to France for arms.

1753

Carl Linnaeus, the famed Swedish botanist, physician, and zoologist, officially names the species *Cannabis sativa* in his book *Species Plantarum, a* work widely acknowledged as the first comprehensive attempt at botanical nomenclature.

1798

French soldiers, sent to conquer Egypt, learn to eat hashish from the locals while in-country, and then return home with some fragrant souvenirs and a taste for more. Upon learning of this new practice, Napoleon attempts to ban hashish entirely in France via an all-out prohibition on possession, sale, and use, but the practice quickly spreads throughout Europe anyway.

1890

Queen Victoria of England uses cannabis to treat her menstrual pain. "When pure and administered carefully," Sir J. Russell Reynolds, her personal physician, wrote in the first-ever issue of the British medical journal *The Lancet*, "it is one of the most valuable medicines we possess."

1910s

Following the Mexican Revolution of 1910, the United States experienced a large wave of Mexican immigration, including many who brought their pot-smoking ways with them when seeking refuge from the war. Once tied to this largely unpopular population influx, the herb became a convenient target for already xenophobic Americans living along the border, who linked *marihuana* to murder and insanity, and began passing laws against it decades before the feds got involved.

1935

The Chinese government enacts a ban against cannabis cultivation.

1937

As the first commissioner of the Federal Bureau of Narcotics, Harry J. Anslinger launched America's original War on Marijuana by portraying pot as an unqualified menace to society. He invented fantastic descriptions of weed-crazed Negroes on grass-fueled killing sprees, who paused in their rampaging only long enough to seduce white women with reefer sticks, then used these and equally lurid tales to scare the populace into compliance with his quixotic attempt to eradicate *marihuana*.

Eventually, Anslinger convinced Congress to enact the Marihuana Tax Stamp Act of 1937, which didn't make cannabis illegal so much as levy taxes on its sale so high that nobody could afford to legally sell it. We've been compounding his folly ever since.

1942

Produced and distributed by the US Department of Agriculture during World War II, *Hemp for Victory* is a classic propaganda film extolling the virtues of marijuana's non-psychoactive cousin, including a laudatory history of hemp, a chronicling of its many uses, and an explanation of why its propagation was so vital to US military interests.

In deference to the War on Weed, the government later denied any such film ever existed, until dogged cannabis researcher and *The Emperor Wears No Clothes* author Jack Herer unearthed a copy in the Library of Congress and proved them wrong.

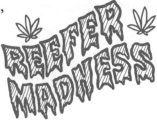

1944

New York City mayor Fiorello La Guardia releases the findings of a blue-ribbon panel tasked with making a full scientific investigation of marijuana based on all previous research, plus their own experiments. Issued as *The La Guardia Report*, the landmark paper includes the endorsement of the prestigious New

York Academy of Medicine, which helped supply the panel with eminent doctors, psychiatrists, psychologists, pharmacologists, chemists, and sociologists.

"Marijuana, like alcohol, does not alter the basic personality," the report concludes. "Marijuana does not of itself produce antisocial behavior. There is no evidence to suggest that the continued use of marijuana is a stepping-stone to the use of opiates. Prolonged use of the drug does not lead to physical, mental, or moral degeneration, nor is there any evidence of any permanent deleterious effects from its continued use. Quite the contrary, marijuana and its derivatives and allied synthetics have potentially valuable therapeutic applications that merit future investigation." For good measure, the report also affirms that "marijuana is not the determining factor in the commission of major crimes."

1961

The United Nations Single Convention on Narcotic Drugs requires all signatories to ban marijuana cultivation, distribution, and use.

1970

Public interest attorney Keith Stroup founds the National Organization for the Reform of Marijuana Laws (NORML) in Washington, DC, now the nation's oldest and largest organization dedicated to cannabis legalization.

1972

After studying marijuana for two years, US president Richard Nixon's handpicked Shafer Commission returns with a detailed report advising Congress to immediately remove all criminal penalties for cannabis, because "neither the marihuana user nor the drug itself can be said to constitute a danger to public safety." But Tricky Dick decides to trash the report instead. The following year, he creates the Drug Enforcement Administration (DEA) and tasks them with waging an all-out war on weed.

1974

After landmark research funded by the National Institutes of Health (NIH), originally designed to prove that marijuana damages the immune system, ended up showing that THC can inhibit the growth of cancer cells in mice, *The Journal of the National Cancer Institute* publishes an academic paper titled "Anticancer Activity of Cannabinoids." The study's primary authors, naturally, immediately promise to investigate this exciting development further, but then the federal government cuts off their funding, pushes their offending report straight down the memory hole, and moves aggressively to block *all* medical-cannabis research moving forward.

It would take nearly thirty years before Dr. Manuel Guzmán, professor of biochemistry at the University of Madrid, managed to follow up on these experiments, with similar results. In fact, Guzmán found that cannabinoids not only shrink cancerous tumors in mice, but they do so without damaging surrounding tissue.

1975

  Robert Randall, who suffers from severe glaucoma, becomes the first federally legal medical-marijuana patient in America after successfully suing the FDA, the DEA, the National Institute on Drug Abuse (NIDA), the Department of Justice (DoJ), and the Department of Health, Education, and Welfare. The US government thus begins supplying Randall and a handful of other patients with cannabis grown at a federally contracted facility in Mississippi, only to abruptly discontinue the Compassionate Investigational New Drug Program in 1992.

A small number of patients, grandfathered into the program, continue to receive up to 300 pre-rolled marijuana joints from the federal government every month to this day.

1988

Francis Young, an administrative law judge with the DEA, rules that cannabis should be allowed for medical use, after concluding that "marijuana in its natural form is one of the safest therapeutically active substances known to man." But the Reagan administration and the DoJ quickly and effectively move to block this ruling and uphold their total ban on marijuana for any use.

1996

California voters pass Proposition 215, the first statewide medical-marijuana law. For the next fifteen years, medical-marijuana growers, patients, and providers face the daily threat of arrest, armed raids, and imprisonment by the federal government—even if fully in compliance with their own state's laws and guidelines.

Despite these unconscionable attacks, the medical-marijuana movement grows and spreads to dozens more states.

2002

Arriving just after dawn, thirty heavily armed DEA agents raid the medical-marijuana garden of the Wo/Men's Alliance for Medical Marijuana (WAMM), a Santa Cruz, California, collective focused on servicing the seriously ill and those unable to afford medicine. Several WAMM members die as a result of being cut off from their supply. In response, less than two weeks after the DEA raid, WAMM gathers on the steps of city hall, alongside the mayor of Santa Cruz and other local officials, to defiantly distribute free medicine to terminally ill members. Next, WAMM successfully sues the federal government, giving the medical-marijuana movement a major victory against the DEA.

2012

Voters in Colorado and Washington pass marijuana legalization by wide margins, making them the first two US states to allow marijuana for all adults twenty-one and over, including state-licensed commercial cultivation and retail sales.

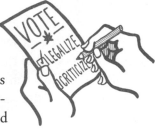

2013

Uruguay passes a government-sponsored bill and becomes the first nation on Earth to fully legalize marijuana cultivation, distribution, and use for all adults. "We are regulating a market that already exists," Uruguayan president José Mujica explained in an interview. "We are trying to regulate and intervene in this market because trafficking is worse than drugs."

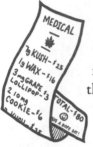

2014

On New Year's Day, Colorado's recreational marijuana stores open for the first time. The author of this book is the eighth person in the state to make a legal purchase and (perhaps) the first to cry a little while asking for a receipt.

2014

On Election Day, voters in Oregon; Alaska; and Washington, DC, pass cannabis legalization initiatives, proving that America's marijuana majority remains ascendant, and revealing the opposition's fear-mongering about legalization as a fraud.

2015

Jamaica's first ever legal ganja plant goes into the ground with the full approval of the justice minister, who sees the creation of a national medical-marijuana system as the first step toward full legalization on the island.

2016

Marijuana legalization becomes a major issue in a US presidential election for the first time.

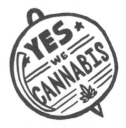

The war on marijuana destroys lives, undermines communities, corrupts the justice system, and costs society billions every year in lost revenue and wasted enforcement resources. On the plus side, however, at least weed remains plentiful and relatively easy to find.

WAR ON WEED: BY THE NUMBERS

- According to the United Nations, more than **150 million** people around the world use marijuana, and the total value of that global marijuana market exceeds **$140 billion**.

- America's marijuana black market is estimated at over **$20 billion** per year, with a significant portion of the profits going to Mexican drug cartels, violent street gangs, and organized crime.

- Marijuana prohibition costs US taxpayers roughly **$20 billion** per year, according to a Harvard-led study, with half that money going to enforcement efforts and half to lost tax revenue.

- From 2001 to 2010, law enforcement made over **8 million** pot busts in the United States alone, a huge factor in America having by far the world's highest incarceration rate. The private, for-profit prison industry now brings in more than **$5 billion** per year.

- Despite using marijuana at the same rate or less than whites, blacks are **four times** as likely to be arrested for marijuana possession.

- More than **200,000 students** have lost federal financial aid because of a drug conviction, including simple possession of marijuana.

- In Colorado's first year of recreational marijuana sales, the state's retailers sold more than **130 metric tons** of cannabis buds and nearly **50 million** units of marijuana-infused edibles, bringing in **$60 million** in tax revenue for the state. In the first five months of 2015, Colorado schools netted **$13.6 million** in tax revenue from legal cannabis. Since legalization, crime rates, unemployment, and traffic fatalities have all gone down.

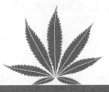

CHAPTER 1

Farm to Pipe

So powerful it can quell grand mal seizures, so gentle you'll never suffer a hangover, cannabis is the closest thing on Earth to a miracle plant. So what could be more fascinating than getting up close and personal with lovely Ms. Mary Jane?

Prior to first meeting Valerie Leveroni Corral, cofounder and director of the Wo/Men's Alliance for Medical Marijuana (WAMM) in Santa Cruz, California, I'd already had the honor and privilege of documenting dozens of different marijuana grows—legal and illegal, indoors and outdoors, organic and hydroponic, one-light closet tents and large "guerrilla gardens" clandestinely planted in remote, difficult-to-access backcountry. But typically I stuck around just long enough to take a guided tour, interview the cultivators, inventory the plants, and sample the goods before heading home to write my story.

Then, in 2010, after seven years working out of *High Times* headquarters in midtown Manhattan, I relocated to Northern California, and took on a new role as the magazine's West Coast editor.

Seeking the true heart and soul of the California cannabis movement, I made WAMM one of my first stops upon reaching the left coast. I'd already heard and read much about the collective's politics—how for twenty years they've focused on low-income, seriously ill patients otherwise unable to afford medicine; how they helped pass America's first statewide medical-marijuana law; and how they survived a DEA raid, then turned around two weeks later and defiantly distributed marijuana to the terminally ill on the steps of city hall—but I had no idea how they managed to plant, tend, and harvest a garden productive enough to supply their hundreds of members with cannabis for an entire year with only a skeleton crew and a small, dedicated team of volunteers.

On the chilly spring morning when I visited WAMM for the first time, the collective's fledgling seedlings were just getting transplanted into five-gallon pots. Valerie put my wife, Elise, and I to work right away, digging holes and mixing soil. She also welcomed us into an amazing community of reefer revolutionaries, and encouraged us to come back for more. So over the next year (and the years to follow) I got to closely follow the crop's natural life cycle—from seed to harvest—for the first time, while making a lot of new, kindhearted friends, learning the art and craft of outdoor cannabis growing, and at long last, getting some dirt under my fingernails.

"Growth is so obvious in the garden—you don't have to wait long to see it," Valerie once told me, explaining that many seriously ill and even terminal patients find the process of producing their own medicine to be highly empowering. "The garden gives us an opportunity to build something bigger than ourselves. That not only helps the healing, it puts us more in touch with the cycles of life."

So let's begin by understanding how the cannabis plant germinates, grows, flowers, and reproduces, and then we'll explore the many ways clever cultivators seek to optimize this process in search of higher potency and heavier harvests.

THE CANNABIS LIFE CYCLE

Like humanity, *Cannabis sativa* is a dioecious species, which means it predominantly produces distinctly male and female organisms, in roughly equal number. Pot is also an annual, meaning individual members of the species complete their entire life cycle in less than one year.

In nature, each plant begins life when a previously dormant seed begins to germinate in early spring. Only the strongest and most viable of these seeds manage to throw off their seed casings, stretch into seedlings, grow into mature plants, and propagate the species. The rest, at some point along that journey, fall by the genetic wayside, helpfully winnowing the herd through natural selection.

Seeds and Clones

Whether dropped naturally in the autumn by a wild pot plant in the far reaches of Afghanistan's rugged Kush mountain range, or carefully placed into a moistened rock-wool cube by a state-licensed marijuana grower in Boulder, Colorado, every genetically distinct cannabis plant on Earth starts as a seed—though like many commercial crops, from bananas and avocados to vanilla and lavender, the vast majority of the marijuana in circulation actually began life as a "clone" or "cutting."

Seedlings grow faster and heartier than these cuttings, but

only after a long, delicate germination period. So most cannabis cultivators opt to start each new crop not from seed but by plucking healthy leaves from the lower branches of a special "mother plant" kept for this purpose, and then replanting those leaves in soil or a medium to take root—a technique that saves weeks of growth time on the front end, and also ensures a genetically uniform set of plants moving forward, which is especially important when trying to manage a tightly packed indoor grow.

Another big advantage of using cuttings is that all your plants will be female (assuming you start with a female "mother plant," of course). Only females produce THC and marijuana's other medicinal and/or psychoactive components in appreciable amounts, so taking clones saves the trouble of waiting for seedlings to show their sex (at about six weeks) and then culling all the males.

Vegetative Growth

Seedlings and clones require a couple of weeks to establish themselves, at which point they "take root," and enter a period of rapid growth. Whether cultivated indoors or out, cannabis will remain in this "vegetative" state—growing taller and wider, and producing a large number of leaves, but not budding—as long as it's exposed to more than twelve hours of light per day.

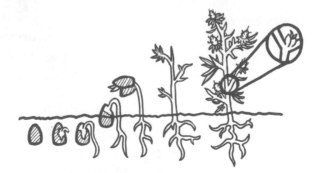

Flowering

As the days grow shorter in the autumn, and in particular when the available daylight dips below twelve hours per day, female cannabis plants begin flowering. At which point, they stop growing significantly taller or wider, instead focusing energy on producing more and larger buds covered in *trichomes*—resinous glands that look like tiny crystals to the naked eye, and like a fluid-filled globe atop a matchstick when magnified.

Male cannabis plants also flower, but unlike females, their flowers don't produce significant amounts of THC-laden resin, so savvy marijuana cultivators either grow all females from clone or, if growing from seed, kill off all their male plants long before they reach maturity. Either way, the resulting all-female crop, if effectively shielded from pollination, will reach maturity without seeds (or sinsemilla, as the technique is commonly known).

Now, as anybody of a certain age can tell you, there's nothing wrong with smoking seeded pot, once you remove the seeds, but it's also, assuredly, less than ideal, because all the unique compounds in cannabis, collectively known as cannabinoids— including the ones that get you high and help prevent Alzheimer's—are predominantly found in the trichomes. And once a formerly virginal female comes in contact with the wind-blown pollen of a male plant, she immediately curtails cannabinoid production in favor of literally "going to seed."

Harvest and Curing

As a female cannabis flower matures, its trichomes change color, starting off clear, turning a translucent milky white, and finally darkening to amber. Harvesting on the early side (translucent trichomes) can limit overall potency but offers a more cerebral, soaring *high*, while waiting until the trichomes turn amber yields a stronger but more sedative *stone*.

Whenever harvest happens, it takes weeks after cutting down a plant to properly dry, trim, and cure its flowers. Start by stripping off the large fan leaves and hanging the buds from their stems in a cool, dark place with steady air circulation for seven to ten days. Trimmed leaves can be saved to make hashish (see page 48), while smokable flowers, once sufficiently dry, are carefully manicured with scissors to remove the smaller, higher-potency "sugar leaves."

From there, the buds must be cured to leech out the last traces of moisture trapped inside—an often overlooked process that actually plays an outsized role in the smokability of the end product.

"It's a lot like the aging of a fine wine," legendary cannabis breeder DJ Short, creator of Blueberry, Old Time Moonshine, and other popular strains, told me once for a *High Times* story. "The benefits of properly cured cannabis include even moisture content and a complete breakdown of chlorophyll, which allows the full, clear expression of taste and aroma to emerge."

Most growers cure buds by carefully stacking as many as possible into an airtight container without damaging them. Over time, trace amounts of moisture inside the buds will evaporate. Periodically opening the container and turning the buds over releases this moisture and allows more to sweat out until the buds are perfectly and evenly dry (usually about a week).

At which point, at long lost, the herb is ready to blaze.

YOU'VE GOT TO HIDE YOUR
LOVE AWAY: HOW PROHIBITION
CHANGED WEED GROWING

Back in the Jazz Age, when pot smoking first achieved international notoriety, there was no such thing as indoor chronic anywhere on Earth, and marijuana was still an import crop in the United States. In those pre-prohibition days, the nation's rather meager supply reached our shores not as a commercial product per se, but rather as a friendly camp follower passed around among in-the-know aficionados.

Still legal in most states until the mid-1930s, in part due to its obscurity, the herb counted among its earliest adopters migrant Mexican farmhands, who grew *marihuana* at home and brought it with them when moving north in search of work, and New Orleans's freewheeling jazz musicians, who got their hands on Caribbean-grown ganja from sailors freshly arrived at the city's bustling port. Both groups eagerly spread the practice to outsiders they encountered, but it was the jazz cats who turned *gage* into a national phenomenon, literally scattering cannabis seeds far and wide during their travels on the music circuit, and figuratively doing the same by inserting sly, appreciative references to reefer into their recordings and radio appearances.

As Cab Calloway sang in his 1933 hit "Reefer Man," which doubled as a somewhat impractical guide to finding a pot dealer, "If he trades you dimes for nickels, and calls watermelons pickles," he's probably the reefer man.

Of course, no good turn goes unpunished in America, especially if you're black or Mexican, and so once the establishment caught a whiff of this fragrant new cultural trend, the government and the media started cooking up a scare campaign designed to turn *marihuana* into a terrifying menace. Then they used the resulting public panic as a way to seek authoritarian control over both the cannabis plant and the undesirable people consuming it.

"I consider marijuana the worst of all narcotics, far worse than the use of morphine or cocaine," Judge John Foster Symes

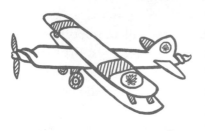

declared in 1937 while sentencing Samuel Caldwell, the first person arrested under federal marijuana prohibition, to four years of hard labor for dealing two joints in the lobby of a seedy Denver hotel. "Marijuana destroys life itself. I have no sympathy with those who sell this weed. The government is going to enforce this new law to the letter."

Maybe so, but soon enough, a loosely knit black market sprouted up to supply marijuana to the masses despite this new prohibition, headed by an iconoclastic, decentralized corps of small-time international pot smugglers—a system that remained largely in place until 1973, when Richard Nixon created the DEA, and tasked them with stopping the steady flow of foreign weed into the United States.

Within a few years of that first salvo in the modern War on Drugs, imported herb became expensive and hard to score, due to massive interdiction efforts on the borders and the long prison sentences handed out to those who got caught. Eventually, the little guys wouldn't take the risk anymore, and the real criminals quickly discovered that cocaine brought in much higher profits, and so a market vacuum opened that didn't make people stop smoking pot but did inspire large numbers of them to start experimenting with growing their own.

A lot of high-paying jobs were thus created right here at home by transforming the nation's underground marijuana supply line from an import business into a cottage industry. Which made everyone happy, except the smugglers, and the human paraquats running the DEA, who decided to respond to the scourge of people growing unauthorized plants on their own land, or out in the middle of nowhere, by recruiting a bunch of combat helicopter pilots who were battle-hardened in Vietnam and ordering them to fly sorties all over the country, seeking out marijuana plantations from the air and terminating them with extreme prejudice.

And so, in a classic case of unintended consequences, the DEA basically invented indoor marijuana growing. Not by secretly designing and selling the high-intensity discharge lights required to cultivate full-potency pot indoors (unless you believe some seriously *far-out* conspiracy theories) but simply by creating a set of incentives that unleashed a massive wave of American ingenuity on the question of how to transform cannabis into a hothouse flower.

As a result, once again, our nation's incredibly resourceful cannabis community went a little further underground. In many cases *literally* underground, as a large, unfinished basement is often the ideal place to grow indoor marijuana away from the prying eyes of Big Government's black helicopters. At least, that was the case ten years ago, when even the world's most skilled indoor cannabis cultivators typically helmed operations of just a dozen 1,000-watt lights, most often concealed within their own homes. Nowadays, of course, state-licensed marijuana cultivation facilities can be truly industrial-size operations, employing dozens of people and producing hundreds of pounds of usable bud or more per month.

A few days before Colorado's recreational pot stores opened to the public for the first time on January 1, 2014, I visited one such operation, the awe-inspiring cultivation facility of Denver's Medicine Man, which ranks among the state's leading marijuana dispensaries. Seeking background for a trilogy of VICE articles (*Tomorrow, I'm going to buy legal weed; I just bought legal weed; I just smoked legal weed*), I took a guided tour of a grow room the size, scale, and professionalism of which I could have scarcely dreamed possible just a few years earlier.

Medicine Man features a sleek, modern retail space up front, with 40,000 square feet of dedicated cultivation and processing space housed in the same building—albeit behind locked and heavily secured doors. Andy Williams, Medicine Man's principal owner, told me he'd rather not put a number on the amount of marijuana they harvest on-site every month, lest any nefarious characters start to get ideas, but let's just say it's more than enough to make Snoop Dogg blush.

Andy, however, never blushes. He's a former military officer and aerospace executive with a hard nose for business and an unshakable determination to build his family-run enterprise into an industry leader. Only he doesn't smoke pot, and doesn't know a thing about growing it. So he leaves all that to his green-thumbed brother Pete.

"People think it takes a lone mystical grower, some guru, to produce top-grade marijuana," Pete, who most certainly does get high on his own supply, told me, "but it doesn't. It takes a standard operating procedure."

Of course, Pete didn't start from scratch when designing and building Medicine Man's state-of-the-art cultivation system, but rather took a scientific approach to scaling up and refining a series of techniques and procedures long developed by underground growers. Because whether you're cultivating just four illicit plants in a closet for head stash and extra cash, or tending to an "indoor acre" of fully legal commercial cannabis, the objective remains the same: to yield the largest amount of high-quality marijuana possible, as quickly and efficiently as possible.

Unfortunately, many of the methods developed to meet this goal resemble the agribusiness world of monocropping and factory farming far more than I'd like to admit, with the added drag of running all those energy-intense grow lights eighteen to twenty-four hours a day. Which means the dirty little secret of the cannabis industry is that a product typically identified with "green values" can have a shockingly high carbon footprint, and other serious environmental consequences, depending on where and how it's grown.

From a purely technical perspective, however, indoor growing offers several clear advantages, which explains why it retains market dominance even in states with fully regulated cultivation. For starters, skilled indoor growers can achieve total mastery of their plants' environment, including consistently providing the optimal temperature, humidity, nutrients, air circulation, and irrigation needed to promote rapid growth. Indoor growers also decide exactly how much artificial sunlight their plants will receive, including when to induce flowering by lowering the photoperiod below twelve hours per day. So while outdoor gardens produce only one harvest each year (typically in late September/early October), indoor growers usually start flowering their plants a mere two to four weeks after they take root as clones, with the entire clone-to-harvest cycle taking just ninety days or so.

My good friend and cannabis colleague Danny Danko, senior cultivation editor at *High Times*, believes that, closely examined, indoor marijuana isn't just a different *process* from outdoor, it's in many ways a different product.

"Marijuana flowers grown indoors tend to be denser than their outdoor counterparts, and because people tend to grow less indoors than outside, the quality of the trimming is usually better too, with less leaf material present. This means the bud-to-leaf ratio tends to be higher for indoor pot, making it taste better (less harsh leaf taste) and burn better," Danny asserts.

From my first days at the magazine, Danny, who grew a lot

of pot plants before he ever started writing about it, patiently guided me through the intricacies of indoor cultivation, helping me understand how a group of outlaws and outcasts took the lemons handed them by the DEA and turned them into Super Lemon Haze (and White Widow, and a thousand other marijuana varieties specially bred to thrive when hidden away in the attic, like something out of *Jane Eyre*).

Indoor growers also learned to greatly increase overall production by dividing their cultivation space into separate vegetative and flowering areas, so that when one set of plants is ready to harvest, another set is done with the vegetative state and big enough to move into the flowering room. In addition to greatly boosting an operation's aggregate yield over the course of the year, such "perpetual harvest" setups also assure harvests of a manageable size, on a set schedule that allows time to dry, trim, and cure each batch before the next one's ready.

BETTER KNOW YOUR CANNABINOIDS: A PRIMER ON POT'S UNIQUE COMPOUNDS

Ever since the discovery of the body's natural endocannabinoid system in the late 1980s, we've come to understand that the brain makes its own "endogenous" cannabinoids naturally, and that these compounds play a critical role in regulating many of the body's most basic functions.

"The endogenous cannabinoid system, named after the plant that led to its discovery, is perhaps the most important physiologic system involved in establishing and maintaining human health," writes Dr. Dustin Sulak, a leading researcher and practitioner of what some have dubbed cannabinopathic medicine. "Endocannabinoids and their receptors are found throughout the body: in the brain, organs, connective tissues, glands, and immune cells. In each tissue, the cannabinoid system performs different tasks, but the goal is always the same: homeostasis, the maintenance of a stable internal environment despite fluctuations in the external environment."

These receptors not only work with the body's natural endocannabinoids, they also fit the pot plant's cannabinoids like a lock fits a key. Which explains how one all-natural botanical can provide so many seemingly unrelated health benefits (see page 94).

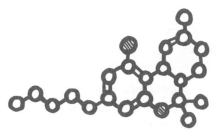

While THC is by far the best known and most psychoactive of cannabis's unique chemical compounds, there's also CBD, CBN, CBG, THC-A, and eighty other cannabinoids worth knowing, as each offers distinct, profound medicinal benefits. Unfortunately, while there's definitely good reason to believe that a lack of natural endocannabinoids may be the underlying cause of a wide variety of serious health problems, and consuming cannabis medicinally could potentially bring those systems back into balance, due to the government's pervasive anti-marijuana ideology, we're decades behind in researching cannabinoids' role in treating illness and maintaining wellness.

One thing we do know for certain, despite the federal government's consistent "crop blocking" of medical-marijuana research, is that if you disrupt the body's natural cannabinoid system, things quickly go haywire. Because that's exactly what happened when Big Pharma tested Rimonabant, an anti-obesity drug designed to create a kind of "reverse munchies" by preventing cannabinoids from reaching their receptors. (The drug also had the related side effect of making it impossible to get high no matter how much weed you smoked.) While those enrolled in a planned thirty-three-month study of Rimonabant *did* report lower overall appetite when taking the drug, they also demonstrated an increased suicide risk so profound the study was abandoned after little more than a year—and four suicides.

"Patients taking Rimonabant reported feeling severely depressed and having serious thoughts about committing suicide," *Psychology Today* reported. "It was as though the patients had lost their ability to experience pleasure . . . [which] tells neuroscientists that our endogenous marijuana system is normally involved, either directly or indirectly, in controlling our mood and allowing us to experience pleasure; antagonizing the actions of this chemical in the brain leads to depression with possibly dangerous consequences."

Think about it this way: A small addition of iodine to your diet can prevent otherwise terribly debilitating goiter, and British sailors once carried limes on board (and earned the nickname limeys) to avoid getting scurvy while at sea, but we didn't always know how to prevent those conditions. So how many people are suffering needlessly right now for want of a small daily cannabinoid supplement?

Fortunately, most retail cannabis shops display THC and CBD percentages for the strains they sell, and in the very near future, a whole range of *nutraceuticals* will be widely available, offering tailored cannabinoid blends designed to boost specific functions in the body.

For now, here's a primer on the key compounds to keep in mind.

THC

If you know only one cannabinoid, it's definitely THC, and with good reason. Other cannabinoids have medicinal/therapeutic properties, after all, but none of them make music sound better, and ice cream taste better, like THC. One of the safest therapeutic substances known to man, it's proven to help treat and prevent cancer, Alzheimer's, and many other serious conditions. Also, it can also get you high as fuck.

THC-A

A precursor, acidic form of the THC that gets you high as fuck, THC-A is non-psychoactive and found in abundance in freshly harvested cannabis. THC-A must be heated to the point of decarboxylation (around 200 degrees Fahrenheit) before it converts into THC, which explains why you can't just eat a raw bud to get high. While THC-A doesn't get you blazed, it does offer many of the benefits of THC, including anti-inflammatory, anti-tumor, and anti-spasmodic properties.

Cannabidiol (CBD)

Cannabidiol has been on the radar of both the pharmaceutical industry and the medical-marijuana community for decades. But it remained a rather obscure little molecule until CNN's chief medical correspondent Dr. Sanjay Gupta introduced the world to Charlotte Figi—a nine-year-old girl who suffered three hundred grand mal seizures every week before non-psychoactive, CBD-rich cannabis oil proved over 99 percent effective in stopping them.

Also a safe, highly effective treatment for pain, insomnia, nausea, anxiety, spasticity, MS, Alzheimer's, cancer, and a host of other serious conditions, CBD not only doesn't get you high, it actually works to temper the high of THC, which explains why underground cannabis breeders largely unwittingly bred it out of the cannabis gene pool during prohibition.

In 2010, Project CBD formed to address this problem, bringing together physicians, scientists, growers, cannabis-testing laboratories, patients, and retailers interested in learning more about CBD's medical potential, including by actively seeking out the world's few remaining CBD-rich strains and helping to breed new ones. Ever since, demand for CBD has grown steadily, particularly among pediatric patients. To access the best science-based information regarding CBD, please visit: projectcbd.org.

Cannabinol (CBN)

An oxidation product of THC, CBN is less psychoactive than its antecedent, with a strongly sedative effect. So if you've ever smoked weed that put you right to sleep, a high CBN profile could be the reason — which is great if you're an insomniac, and terrible if you're at a Rush concert. Most times CBN forms when you let your pot sit around for a few weeks in a baggie or expose it to heat, light, or the air for prolonged periods (instead of storing it properly in an airtight jar kept in a cool, dark place). It can also happen if you cook your edibles too long or at too high of a temperature.

Cannabichromene (CBC)

Rarely found in commercially available cannabis except in trace amounts, CBC is non-psychoactive, with sedative, antianxiety properties. Research has shown strong antidepressant effects, and CBC has also been proven to enhance the pain-relief properties of THC.

Cannabigerol (CBG)

Nonpsychoactive and commonly found in low levels (less than 1 percent) in most cannabis samples, CBG has demonstrated pain relief, antibiotic, and anti-inflammatory benefits. It also reduces intraocular pressure, associated with glaucoma.

THE NOSE KNOWS: GIVING WEED THE SMELL TEST

In these decidedly heady days of post-prohibition euphoria, when dedicated cannabis analytical laboratories report on a particular bud's exact percentage of THC prior to it ever reaching your bong, and enterprising geneticists work tirelessly on mapping the genome sequence of popular pot strains with an eye toward creating powerful new medicines, it's easy to forget that not so long ago, those tasked with assessing a particular herbal specimen's potency relied largely on the old adage "the nose knows."

In fact, one of the most intriguing characters I've encountered in my marijuana travels is known simply as "The Nose." Employed for many years as a cannabis broker, middle-manning deals between growers and dealers, he regularly sets the price on major transactions with nothing more authoritative than his olfactory sense and his reputation. But if THC, the cannabis plant's primary psychoactive component, is odorless, how can The Nose really know anything?

The answer lies in a set of compounds called *terpenoids* (or terpenes), which provide a strain's particular aroma. Produced within the plant's trichomes, right alongside cannabinoids like THC and CBD, more than two hundred different terpenoids have been identified in cannabis, and according to physician and researcher Dr. Ethan Russo, they not only smell strongest in herb of the highest potency, they also play an important role in what he calls marijuana's "entourage effect."

In a 2011 paper published by the prestigious *British Journal of Pharmacology*, Russo described these "phytocannabinoid-terpenoid entourage effects," or, in layman's terms, the way compounds wholly unique to cannabis (cannabinoids) work best in the presence of various terpenes, which can be found in marijuana and a wide variety of other plants. So if The Nose detects a powerful blast of pine when lowering his delicate instrument into a bag of Sour Diesel, for example, he knows that particular batch was grown to its full potential. He can't smell the THC, but any bud pumping out that much alpha-Pinene—the terpenoid responsible for the pine smell—has surely been expertly grown, and harvested at or near the strain's peak potency.

Naturally, since pot that smells amazing fetches a premium, cannabis breeders constantly seek to bring out the plant's natural terpenoids when creating new varieties. This has led to vast differences in terpenoid profile, which explains why different strains excel at treating different ailments, despite largely relying on the same or similar blends of THC and CBD as the primary therapeutic agents. It also explains why some people like the high of a particular strain so much they smoke it exclusively.

To help you find your flavor, here's the basics on the most common terpenes found in cannabis, including some common strains that fit the profile.

ALPHA-PINENE, also found in pine needles, works as a powerful bronchodilator. So the same way your lungs feel clean and expanded after a brisk walk through the pines, cannabis rich in alpha-Pinene can positively affect conditions like asthma and fatigue. Alpha-Pinene also boasts antibacterial and antibiotic properties.

Found in: Blue Dream, Sour Diesel

LIMONENE, also found in lemons, improves mood, relieves heartburn and gastrointestinal reflux, helps lower cholesterol, and offers other heart-healthy benefits. In lab experiments, limonene has demonstrated anti-cancer properties, and has antimicrobial effects that combat pathogenic bacteria.

Found in: OG Kush, Lemon Haze

MYRCENE, also found in the flowers of the hops vine, provides anti-inflammatory benefits and works as a sedative. According to Dr. Ethan Russo, likely the first scientist to use the term "couch lock" in the *British Journal of Pharmacology*: "Myrcene acted as a muscle relaxant in mice, and potentiated barbiturate sleep time at high doses. . . . It may produce the 'couch-lock' phenomenon of certain chemotypes that is alternatively decried or appreciated by recreational cannabis consumers."

Found in: Purple Kush, Super Silver Haze

LINALOOL, also found in lavender, helps regulate serotonin neurotransmission, eases anxiety, and counters insomnia. Linalool is also a strong anticonvulsant with an antidepressant effect.

Found in: Kush Daddy, Fire OG

BETA-CARYOPHYLLENE, also found in black pepper, is anti-inflammatory, but unlike many other anti-inflammatories, it protects the stomach lining rather than damaging it. It's used for treating certain ulcers and irritable bowels.

Found in: Chem Dawg, Trainwreck

HEMP, HEMP, HOORAY

Smoke enough herb, and at some point, somebody will start enthusiastically evangelizing hemp, including telling you how marijuana's straitlaced, non-psychoactive cousin produces fiber of incredible strength and versatility, how the plant's seed oil is the world's most nutritionally complete single food source, and how a drought-resistant crop that thrives without pesticides and fertilizers has the potential to replace drilling, logging, mining, monoculture corn farming, plastics, energy exploration, and countless other environmentally destructive industries.

Unfortunately, hemp got lumped in with marijuana back in 1937 when the United States first passed federal weed prohibition, and the hardworking no-high plant with the potential to disrupt many modern industries has faced an uphill climb ever since. Lately, however, along with the legalization of cannabis, there's been a welcome move toward re-legalizing hemp as well.

In 2014, the US Congress passed a Farm Bill that included an amendment allowing universities and state agriculture departments to "experiment" with hemp in any state with a law approving such production, opening the door for America's first fully legal crop since at least World War II.

But now that we've finally started coming to our senses, the question becomes, *Can hemp* really *save the world?*

To separate the weed from the chaff, so to speak, I spoke with author and NPR contributor Doug Fine for a VICE article entitled "The Great Hemp Experiment Begins." In his delightful and well-informed book *Hemp Bound*, Fine, a self-described "comedic investigative journalist" (and author of the bestseller *Farewell, My Subaru*) travels the globe to examine the green shoots of the emerging worldwide hemp industry, and reports back on an agricultural/industrial revolution in the making that may indeed be humanity's saving grace.

"Utilized correctly, hemp could have a transformative impact on the future of humanity, including climate mitigation and—ultimately—freedom from fossil fuels," Fine told me. "In just a few years, we won't be discussing if hemp's going to be a massive industry, because the facts on the ground show the Canadian hemp seed oil industry growing 20 percent this year [2014], to nearly $1 billion."

Perhaps someday I'll write a book called *How to Not Smoke Pot (Properly)* that will explain in detail how hemp can feed the world, free us from fossil fuels, and restore our environment, but in the meantime, I'd highly recommend picking up a copy of *Hemp Bound* if you want to know more. Otherwise, given the title and mandate of this book, I'll simply close the subject by asserting that anyone who gives you hemp to smoke (defined by the government as having less than 0.3 percent THC) is not your friend.

INDICA VERSUS SATIVA

Most botanists believe cannabis originated as a wild flowering herb somewhere in western Asia and later split into two subspecies as it began migrating across the globe many thousands of years ago, with *Cannabis sativa* flourishing in equatorial regions, and *Cannabis indica* taking root in higher elevations.

Taxonomists began making distinctions between the two at least as far back as the eighteenth century, based on their differing growth characteristics. *Sativa*s are tall and lanky with thin leaves and mature slowly, yielding wispy buds prized for their uplifting, cerebral effects—making them ideal for mood elevation and cognitive enhancement. *Indica*s are short and squat with thick leaves, and mature quickly, yielding dense, resinous buds that offer a sedative body high that's ideal for treating chronic pain and achieving "couch lock."

Adaptation to vastly different climates caused the original split between *sativa*s and *indica*s, but selective breeding played a crucial role in just *how* different the two subspecies then became, to the point that, grown side by side, few neophytes would believe they're the same species if not for their distinctive leaves.

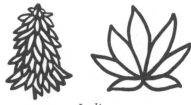

Indica

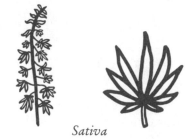

Sativa

That's because *indica*s, native to southern Asia and the Indian subcontinent (Afghanistan, Pakistan, India, Tibet, Nepal), have been bred for millennia to quickly produce fat, trichome-coated buds, as that's the ideal starting material for hash making, a tradition that dates back untold generations in those regions (see page 48). In the equatorial regions where *sativa*s grow, meanwhile, smoking cannabis flowers is and was far more common.

Mexican immigrants first began importing purebred *sativa* strains into America in the early 1900s, and *marihuana*, as the plant soon became derisively known in the press, would remain an imported *sativa* crop in the United States until President Richard M. Nixon created the DEA in 1974 and tasked them with closing America's borders to weed. Which made those much-loved imports much more expensive and way harder to score.

Naturally, countless cannabis enthusiasts of the era tried planting the plentiful seeds that came free in every bag of the most popular strains on the market, including landrace *sativas* from Mexico (Acapulco Gold), Colombia (Punta Roja), Hawaii (Maui Wowie), and Thailand (Thai Stick), only to discover that such equatorial varieties grew poorly outside their home climates. And so, it wasn't until wandering longhairs started returning home from the so-called Hippie Trail with seeds for a new kind of plant—one acclimated to the mountainous regions of Nepal, India, and Pakistan—that the modern era of marijuana breeding truly began.

These new *indica* varieties, like Hash Plant and Afghani, thrived in Northern California, especially once crossbred with more familiar *sativa* varieties to produce amazingly potent best-of-both-worlds hybrids, such as Northern Lights and William's Wonder. By combining the fragrant aroma, smooth smoke, and clear, soaring high of *sativas* with the dense buds, rapid growth cycle, and heavy harvest of *indicas*, these first-generation hybrids transformed cannabis cultivation forever, putting the means of pot production in pretty much everyone's hands, providing you had a place to grow and the gumption to go for it.

Today, almost every strain available, both in the legal marketplace and underground, is a hybrid, though some lean far more in one direction or the other. The judging committee at the *High Times* Cannabis Cup, for instance, allows any strain with 70 percent or more *indica* or *sativa* genetics to compete under those classifications, with the rest categorized as hybrids.

CANNABIS STRAINS: WHAT'S IN A NAME?

That which we call a rose, by any other name would smell as sweet.
—WILLIAM SHAKESPEARE,
ROMEO AND JULIET (ACT 2, SCENE 2)

Shakespeare's right in that what we call a flower has no effect on its aroma, but when it comes to cannabis, the words that signify a particular bud do often offer important clues to not just how it smells but also how it smokes. So where do all those crazy strain names come from anyway?

Well, just like with roses, whoever successfully breeds a new weed strain gets to name it. In theory, that happens every time two unique varieties are crossed, but in practice, only the most successful of these hybrids will grow popular enough for the genetic line to earn a place in the pot pantheon as a distinct new breed. The rest are just mutts.

The tradition of breeding cannabis for desirable traits, meanwhile, is perhaps as old as agriculture itself, and began, likely in western China, when formerly wild-growing weed was first bred into a "landrace" strain—meaning a domesticated, locally adapted variety of the plant. In time, herb farmers worldwide—from the Kush mountains of Afghanistan to the fetid jungles of South America—would develop their own landrace strains, which later served as the genetic building blocks upon which all our popular modern hybrids have been built.

Some landraces (like Kush, Durban, and Afghani) still show up in the names of popular strains, but most hybrids take their moniker from a combination of their attributes and their more direct lineage. For example, Purple Diesel is a hybrid strain with buds that turn purple at harvest. It's descended from the popular Sour Diesel strain (named for its pungent petrol aroma and tart taste) and "Pre-98" Bubba Kush (as opposed to supposedly inferior Bubba Kush that started circulating under that name in 1998). Of course, if you *really* delve into those genetics, you'll find the exact origins of both Sour Diesel and Bubba Kush remain murky—a rather common condition, given the clandestine nature of marijuana breeding back in those days.

Needless to say, this all gets *even more confusing* the further down the rabbit hole you go, and that's *before* you start getting stoned.

🌿 PRO TIP 🌿

SORTING OUT

MARIJUANA STRAINS

"I only smoke O.G. Kush—unless I'm in New York, then it's Sour D."
—B-REAL OF CYPRESS HILL, *LA WEEKLY*

"No matter how much I liked it, I could never say to someone, 'I'd like some Maui Wowie.' I would be so mortified to say that to someone. The high could never compensate."
—JOHN WATERS, *HIGH TIMES*

FROM HASHISH TO DABS:
CLASSIC CONCENTRATIONS

For thousands of years, cannabis cultivators have been concentrating their raw plant material into a more potent, more portable form called hashish, and throughout that long, storied history, they've managed to consistently refine not just the end product but also the processes by which hashish is made and consumed.

In the earliest hash-making traditions, in Morocco, Nepal, India, and elsewhere along the old Spice Road, growers simply wandered through their vast cannabis gardens at harvest time, gathering resin from the buds by hand. According to legend, the finest grade (the "first press," if you will) of this product was collected by a naked virgin sent out into the fields to rub against the herb until too intoxicated from transdermal absorption to continue. (Note: Pot growers, then and now, have a lot of time on their hands to make up stories.)

As you can imagine, carefully hand-collected resin (extra-virgin or otherwise) yields a potent, floral, highly refined product, but it's also a purely artisan endeavor. So when a taste for hashish started to spread around the world starting in the late 1700s, enterprising Moroccan growers developed the sieve method to keep up with rising demand, which involves pushing dried buds through fine woven silk to separate their THC-laden trichomes from surrounding plant matter. Anyone who's ever visited an Amsterdam coffee shop and ordered off the import hash menu knows the distinct, spicy aroma and subtle, exotic high of such hashish, still made today by the same sieve method.

I say *subtle* high because while separating the trichomes from the rest of the plant most assuredly means concentrating the herb's active ingredients, Amsterdam's best import hash still tops out at around 35 percent THC, since the buds used to make it aren't nearly as potent as what you'll find on the shelves in Denver or Seattle. Moroccan hash also has a relatively high CBD profile, which makes for a really mellow, anxiety-free type of high. In fact, medical researchers first got interested in CBD as a potentially useful therapeutic agent when a small group of MS patients shared their stories on the Internet, after discovering that their symptoms almost magically abated whenever they visited Amsterdam's coffee shops (which back then offered far more hashish than raw buds), even if they also smoked pot at home.

Oil and Water

The next major innovation in hashish came when some crafty cannabis grower realized that the plant's trichomes, which contain its THC, CBD, and other cannabinoids, are oil-based, while the vegetative matter they cling to (buds and leaves) is water-based. And since oil and water don't mix, you can easily separate the trichomes by submerging the plant matter in clean water and agitating it. Then pour the water through a series of screens designed to collect different-sized trichomes, and *voilà*—you've got several grades of hashish, each typically purer and more potent than traditionally sieved hash.

Of course, when rating hashish, purity and potency aren't the only qualifications worth considering. Just as wine critics rarely mention a particular vintage's alcohol-by-volume percentage, and most people prefer drinking beer to grain alcohol, it's a mistake to confuse "the world's strongest cannabis" for "the best cannabis for me." Personally, I enjoy both kinds of hashish and in an ideal world would have a bit of both on hand at all times—Moroccan-style imports for their depth of flavor, their proud lineage, and the CBD-rich endless groove state they imbue, and "water hash" for its clear taste, smooth smoke, and soaring high.

The most stellar water hash I ever sampled originated on a ganja farm that I profiled several times for *High Times*. Based on their eco-friendly, small-scale, communal approach to commercial cannabis cultivation, I dubbed the place "Weeditopia," a reference to Ernest Callenbach's 1975 cult-classic novel *Ecotopia*, in which Northern California, Oregon, and Washington break off from the United States and form an independent republic based on living in harmony with the natural environment.

The book opens twenty years after the split, when a journalist from New York City becomes the first American to visit Ecotopia since their war of independence, and ends up going native. As a New Yorker long accustomed to looking over my shoulder every time I lit up a joint, I could certainly relate. In fact, after my first few days at Weeditopia, I was already talking about relocating to Northern California, a momentous decision that had a lot more to do with the heady feeling of waking up at dawn to do yoga with a dozen new friends as the morning sun glistens across the most vibrant ganja garden you've ever seen than the fact that they made this amazing hashish. But I'd be lying if I said the hash didn't play a small role.

They made it just once a year at harvest time, when the farm had copious amounts of cannabis "trim" on hand that would otherwise go to waste. The buds, of course, were carefully manicured by hand and saved for smoking, but many other parts of the plant, especially the small leaves near the buds, have appreciable amounts of cannabinoids as well, and can therefore be used for making hash.

An icy-cold mountain stream ran through the property, so rather than setting up a typical system of large buckets and a paint mixer to agitate the trim batch by batch, they used a solar pump to temporarily divert a small portion of the stream and run it through a contractor bag full of trim, followed by a series of micron-size screens specially designed to catch and collect all the trichomes. Then the near-freezing, incredibly pure water poured right back into the stream.

The best grade of this concentrate turned jet-black once dry, with the surface sheen of a moon rock. Widely considered a little too intoxicating for daytime use, the farm crew would gather at sunset after a long, hard day spent leafing and trimming to pass around the hash pipe and swap stories before dinner. To my knowledge, nobody ever lab tested Weeditopia's hashish, but I'm pretty confident it couldn't have been much more than 50 percent THC. Still, I don't remember thinking that what we really needed was something nearly twice as strong.

Something Nearly Twice as Strong

The fastest-growing trend in cannabis culture right now is most definitely *dabbing*, which involves vaporizing an extremely high-potency cannabis concentrate produced by using a chemical solvent (often butane) to extract cannabinoids and terpenes from raw cannabis. The tradition dates back to at least 1970, when a member of the legendary Brotherhood of Eternal Love, a group of outlaw surfer/smugglers who also helped spread LSD worldwide during those heady days, first created "honey oil," a kind of viscous goo that, using modern techniques, can occasionally top 90 percent THC.

Thanks to the brotherhood, honey oil briefly started turning heads on the American market about forty years ago, but then the supply line suddenly dried up. Turns out a cannabis refinery run by the syndicate exploded in Kabul, Afghanistan, halting production and tipping off the US Bureau of Narcotics and Dangerous Drugs to the Brotherhood's smuggling activities. The explosion also offered a lethal foreshadowing of things to come, both in Afghanistan and here in America. Because let's be perfectly clear about this: Outside the hands of qualified professionals, using proper equipment and procedures, butane honey oil (BHO) production is extremely dangerous. People have been killed and severely injured making it incorrectly, or simply living next door to someone who did.

In places like Colorado and Washington State, the government licenses extract makers, who must pass inspection and operate in accordance with strict regulations. But elsewhere the black market pushes this behavior into the shadows, where a teenager with a rice cooker and a working knowledge of *Breaking Bad* suddenly fancies himself a chemist. And even if little Johnny does manage to make a pile of glop without blowing the house up, or spilling toxic chemicals all over himself, do you really want to smoke it?

I don't, and I won't. Hand me pretty much any joint on Earth, and I'll gladly share it with you—especially if you grew it yourself. But please don't be offended if I turn down your homemade BHO. Generally, it's just not my cup of tea. And when I do indulge, I have to know for certain it was made to the highest standards.

Also, as someone heavily invested in seeing cannabis culture flourish, I just don't think blowtorches and 90 percent THC is our best foot forward into the wider world. If that's what you like, then by all means do what you like, but I do worry about people having BHO as their first exposure to the herb. I've seen literal legends of cannabis temporarily reduced to mental rubble by too much BHO taken in too quickly, so I hate to think what that must do to a novice. I'm also turned off by a certain machismo that exists around trying to inhale the biggest dabs of the highest potency, a quest that leads to lots of coughing in the short term, and in time could potentially throw your endocannabinoid system out of whack due to overstimulation.

Anyway, all that said, there's surely no denying the pleasures of the product when properly made and consumed with some moderation. The best dabs hit the palate with a fresh blast of terpenes, followed by an intense, clear high that begins in your forehead and spreads from there like a pool of warmth. Inexperienced users should start small, with a dab about half the size of a grain of rice, consumed while well hydrated and fully seated. And they should wait at least thirty minutes before taking another.

HASH TAGS:
A FIELD GUIDE TO HASHISH OF ALL KINDS

CHARAS—Originally used only in reference to the highest-quality hand-gathered hashish of India, *charas* now describes any fine hashish made by this traditional method.

KIEF—A granular form of hashish made by pushing dry plant matter through a sieve.

BUTANE HONEY OIL (BHO)—A general term for any concentration of cannabis made by dissolving the plant in a chemical solvent (typically butane) and then purging out the solvent.

DAB—A small glob of BHO applied directly to a heat source for personal consumption.

EARWAX—BHO the color and consistency of earwax. Duh . . .

BUDDER—BHO that's whipped into the texture of soft butter.

HONEY BUD—A bud of raw cannabis that's coated with BHO.

WATER HASH—A general term for any concentrate made using water-based extraction techniques.

SHATTER—BHO so brittle it shatters upon contact.

HONEYCOMB—BHO that looks like a honeycomb, with a firm texture.

FLAKE—Budder that's dried out until it flakes apart.

CRUMBLE—Budder with a lighter consistency, so it crumbles at the touch.

ROSIN—A new style of cannabis concentrate made without chemical solvents by applying heat and pressure to lower-potency water hash or raw cannabis buds until a dab-quality oil leaks out.

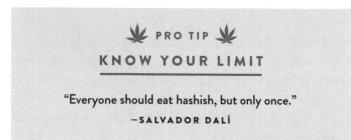

PRO TIP

KNOW YOUR LIMIT

"Everyone should eat hashish, but only once."
—SALVADOR DALÍ

SAFETY MEETING

Since you've read this far, I suppose it's safe to let you know that "safety meeting" has been stoner code for stepping outside to get high for as long as anyone can remember. So definitely don't skip the next one you hear about.

But seriously folks, now that we've learned a fair bit about the plant, and before we move on to exploring how to ingest it properly, I really do want to talk about marijuana safety for a minute, because most people seem to believe either that pot's dangerous (wrong) or that it's harmless (also wrong).

Certainly the facts show "marijuana, in its natural form, is one of the safest therapeutically active substances known to man . . . safer than many foods we commonly consume," according to former DEA chief administrative law judge Francis Young, but still, from driving under the influence to wigging out on pot chocolate to going one toke over the line while smoking superconcentrated dabs, there's definitely more than a few "potholes" to avoid if you want to be a viper.

The good news is that while overdosing on marijuana in any form can be both psychologically alarming and physically debilitating, it will pass in time without any lasting damage to your body or mind. In fact, cannabis is one of the few (if only) psychoactive drugs on Earth with a lethal dose so high as to be essentially theoretical. As Francis Young, the DEA judge, put it:

> *Drugs used in medicine are routinely given what is called an LD-50. The LD-50 rating indicates at what dosage fifty percent of test animals receiving a drug will die as a result of drug induced toxicity. A number of researchers have attempted to determine marijuana's LD-50 rating in test animals, without success. Simply stated, researchers have been unable to give animals enough marijuana to induce death.*

At present it is estimated that marijuana's LD-50 is around 1:20,000 or 1:40,000. In layman terms, this means that in order to induce death a marijuana smoker would have to consume 20,000 to 40,000 times as much marijuana as is contained in one marijuana cigarette. NIDA-supplied marijuana cigarettes weigh approximately .9 grams. A smoker would theoretically have to consume nearly 1,500 pounds of marijuana within about fifteen minutes to induce a lethal response.

So to be safe, never roll a joint that weighs significantly more than 1,000 pounds unless sharing it with several friends. And more seriously, don't ever get behind the wheel of an automobile while dangerously impaired—on anything.

Unfortunately, unlike with alcohol, where a blood alcohol test provides a reasonably accurate gauge of impairment, the science surrounding stoned driving is complex, and confusing—as I explained in a VICE *Motherboard* article called, fittingly, "The Confusing Science of Stoned Driving." For example, a widely reported meta-analysis published in the *British Medical Journal* in 2012 found that marijuana use within one hour of driving nearly doubles the risk of a serious automobile accident. But a later review in the journal *Accident Analysis and Prevention* claimed those findings were overblown, likening increased risk to the use of antihistamines or penicillin.

Then in 2015, the *Washington Post* reported that "a new study from the National Highway Traffic Safety Administration finds that drivers who use marijuana are at a significantly lower risk for a crash than drivers who use alcohol. And after adjusting for age, gender, race and alcohol use, drivers who tested positive for marijuana were no more likely to crash than who had not used any drugs or alcohol prior to driving."

Meanwhile, traffic fatalities seem to drop after states approve medical marijuana, or outright legalization.

"Specifically, we find that traffic fatalities fall by nearly 9 percent after the legalization of medical marijuana," University of Colorado professor Daniel Rees and Montana State University assistant professor D. Mark Anderson concluded in 2011, research results that may sound counterintuitive at first, but actually reflect the one data point that holds steady across all the research: drunk drivers are far more dangerous than stoned drivers, with alcohol use increasing accident risk seventeenfold, according to the US Department of Transportation's National Highway Traffic Safety Administration.

So no, getting high most certainly *doesn't* make you a better or safer driver, it's just that if some people drive stoned instead of drunk, that's a net gain. In any event, always wait at least two hours after smoking weed before driving, and encourage others to be equally responsible. Also, keep in mind that a moving vehicle is one of the easiest places to get arrested for weed, whether or not you live in a state where it's legal to light up at home.

So why risk it?

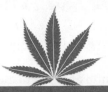

CHAPTER 2

User Guide

*Learn to acquire, assess, appreciate, and
consume cannabis properly, and then
get high with a little help from your
friends.*

When I clocked in for my first day of work at *High Times*
magazine in 2002, I was already long accustomed to smoking
herb on the daily, and yet I understood surprisingly little about
the plant I so deeply revered. As a history buff and amateur
know-it-all, I had a decent grasp of pot politics and the long,
sordid tale of how a highly beneficial plant became an official
menace to society, but when it came to the botany of cannabis,
the science of medical marijuana, and the basics of cultivation,
I didn't know my OG Kush from my Sour Diesel.

To me, marijuana came in exactly two varieties, the com-
pressed brick weed of my youth, imported from Mexico via a
supply chain I'd rather not think about, and "kind buds," which
I generally assumed grew on a remote hillside in Humboldt
County, California.

And so, my sentimental education in all things marijuana largely started when I joined forces with the most esteemed assemblage of weed snobs on the planet, a designation I most assuredly intend (and the *High Times* staff accepts) as a compliment. What followed—from the first time I actually saw a live pot plant growing, to my first trip to Amsterdam for the magazine's annual Cannabis Cup—was a crash course in cannabis like none other. I started out my ten years at *High Times* getting into the trunks of my sources' cars, so I wouldn't be able to incriminate them even if ordered to do so by a judge, and ended it interviewing corporate weed CEOs inside their massive, fully legal marijuana production facilities.

Along the way, I discovered I'm far from the only one who feels a deep, personal connection to this plant. And that whether you try to explain it through chemistry, biology, psychology, sociology, or even shamanism and mysticism, the story of humanity simply can't be told without understanding marijuana—and vice versa.

Something to think about the next time you roll up a joint.

HOW TO ROLL A JOINT (PROPERLY)

My first three years working at *High Times*, I harbored a dark, shameful secret. I couldn't roll a decent joint to save my life—an expression that takes on new meaning when you consider this plant's amazing medicinal properties, and then imagine a nightmare *Twilight Zone*–esque scenario where you're shipwrecked on a deserted tropical island with a whole bale of weed, a case of rolling papers, a thousand lighters, and no way to get faded.

Now, admittedly, it's highly unlikely your own personal moment of being unmasked as a non-roller will be nearly so dramatic as this wholly imagined worst-case scenario, but a crippling fear of facing prejudice, discrimination, and even public ridicule nonetheless keeps millions of people around the world suffering from Joint Rolling Dysfunction Syndrome (JRDS) from coming forward and seeking help. So I'm here on behalf of myself and countless other JRDS survivors to say you don't have to go on living that way. With proper instruction, a positive attitude, and a bit of patience, you too can overcome this debilitating condition and live the life you've always imagined.

So how do you learn to roll a top-notch joint? The same way you get to Carnegie Hall: *Practice, practice, practice . . .*

STEP 1: Assemble at least a gram of cannabis, high-quality rolling papers (raw paper is best, no flavors!), an herb grinder (or scissors in a pinch), a rolling tray, an ashtray, and either cardboard tips to make a filter or a business card you don't mind tearing up.

STEP 2: Block out forty-five minutes to do nothing but learn this one essential skill. Start sober, and make the commitment that you will not smoke weed until you've rolled three perfect joints in a row. Do this alone, with your phone turned off, and preferably on a rainy day sitting next to a window you can occasionally look out of wistfully.

STEP 3: Put on "Kind of Blue" by Miles Davis at moderate volume. Then grind the herb thoroughly, stopping before it becomes powdery. Perhaps the biggest mistake rookie rollers make is either over- or undergrinding their weed. If you keep going until it gets powdery, the flavor will seep out and the joint will burn harsh and quick. And if you leave your buds too chunky, the joint will be hard to roll and burn unevenly.

STEP 4: Watch Danny Danko's "How to Roll a Joint" video on YouTube and do what Danny does. Over and over again, tearing the joint apart each time you finish, and spilling the ground-up weed back into your rolling tray, until you finally get it just right three times in a row without hesitation.

STEP 5: Hold your perfect joint up at arm's length and marvel at it. Feel a sense of self-reliance and self-confidence you've never known before. Then imagine a few scenarios where utilizing your new skill will yield rich rewards, like perhaps meeting a sexy stranger at a party, who pulls you aside in the hallway and asks, seductively, "Hey, do you know how to roll a joint?"

STEP 6: Fire up your masterwork, and—while gazing out the window and listening to Miles—ruminate on the temporal nature of art and existence as the joint burns down to nothing but a resin-stained cardboard filter.

STEP 7: Start learning how to roll a joint when you're already stoned by returning to step 3 and starting over.

HOW TO ROLL A JOINT
IN A WINDSTORM

When it comes to getting high, my focus is always on pragmatic functionality. So if you want to learn how to roll a cross-joint, a windmill, or a tulip, just Google it and go for it, but personally, I only roll two ways: the Danko method detailed above, and a sort-of survivalist technique I learned from a freewheeling cannabis grower we'll call "Jerry," whom I met while engaged in a little field reporting up in Humboldt County.

Although rightly proud of his region's worldwide reputation for growing amazing cannabis, Jerry wanted to make sure I saw something besides greenhouses and planting sheds during my first visit to the Emerald Triangle, so one morning we left at dawn and drove a few hours from his farm to the beach, stopping along the way to take a series of short hikes, during which time I'd sample one of his favorite strains from last year's harvest and offer a few tasting notes. He'd carefully planned all the stops in advance, and expertly rolled all the joints in advance, and (I'm guessing) even paired each joint with each stop (Headband x Waterfall Hike) based on some metric I can only imagine.

It was indeed a lovely, lovely day. But then, as we stood on a cliff overlooking a rugged stretch of Pacific-coast shoreline, disaster loomed, when Jerry realized he'd forgotten to roll something up for the grand finale. We were a long way from our vehicle, but between us scrounged up a rolling paper and a nice dank bud of organic, sun-grown Blackberry Kush. The wind was blowing strong and steady in our faces, and there was absolutely nothing nearby to duck behind.

What happened next (as they say in those cheesy Facebook posts) amazed me. And I've used this same simple hack myself countless times since, in situations ranging from hayrides to softball games.

STEP 1: If right-handed, put a joint's worth of bud in the palm of your left hand.

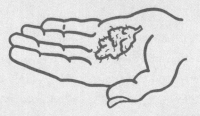

STEP 2: Take out a rolling paper and hold it in your mouth until you need it, careful not to get it wet.

STEP 3: Use your free hand to grind up the bud in the palm of your "tray" hand, cupping your "tray" hand slightly so that no bud spills out or blows away.

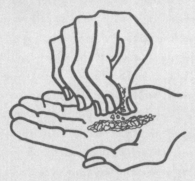

STEP 4: Arrange the ground-up bud in the palm of your hand into the shape of a joint, then lay the rolling paper over the top of it, glue side down.

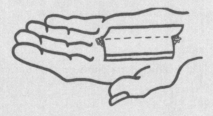

STEP 5: Lay your free hand on top of the rolling paper, and then flip both hands over, so that the rolling paper is now below the bud, and ready to roll. Move quickly from there, and you should have no problem putting together a workable (if imperfect) joint.

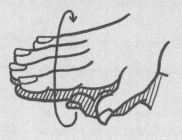

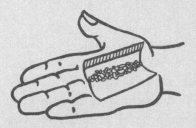

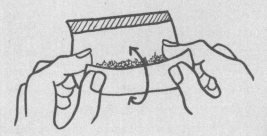

🌿 PRO TIP 🌿

A PROPER HOST CAN
ROLL HER OWN

"Of course I know how to roll a joint."
—MARTHA STEWART TO ANDY COHEN,
WATCH WHAT HAPPENS LIVE

STRAIN SELECTION

With hundreds—if not thousands—of different ganja varieties on offer from cannabis stores, medical-marijuana dispensaries, and black-market dealers around the world, it's necessary to understand the fundamentals of what makes each one distinct before you can properly decide which one's right for you (right now).

From a cultivator's perspective, strain selection involves careful consideration of not just the smell, taste, and high of a particular variety, but also how fast it grows, how much it yields, and what kind of climate best suits its particular genetic makeup. For instance, strains that thrive in a sunny, arid environment may fatally succumb to mold and mildew if planted near a foggy coast. And varieties that develop into towering, bud-laden, twelve-foot-tall monster plants in a greenhouse may prove far too unruly to efficiently cultivate indoors.

So if you ever do decide to grow your own—for medicine, fun, or profit—rather than planting the first seeds you can get your hands on, take the time to carefully research cannabis varieties and breeders to see which strains best suit your needs.

And if you'd rather just geek out on the smell, taste, lineage, and effects of different strains, the best resource available might be an app called Leafly that bills itself formally as "the world's largest cannabis information community," and informally as "the Yelp of marijuana." Click on "Explore Strains," and Leafly will help you find an ideal cannabis variety, edible, concentrate, or topical product based on the precise effect you want, medical condition you'd like to relieve, or even the type of flavors and aromas you enjoy in your herb. The most popular strains have thousands of reviews, as increasing access to retail marijuana has made connoisseurship possible for millions of passionate cannabis lovers who previously got their herb from an outlaw dealer, typically not with a wide array of choices, but as more of a "take it or leave it" proposition.

When I search for a Kush strain near my home in central California, I find twenty-five different varieties available within a short drive, including OG Kush, Master Kush, King's Kush, and Vanilla Kush—an embarrassment of riches that shows just how far we've come in the struggle for safe, legal access to cannabis. At least in some places. When I perform the same Kush search, but change my location to Tulsa, Oklahoma, it predictably yields zero results.

Like Yelp, Leafly and other, similar apps rely on the wisdom of the crowd to rate both cannabis strains and the various stores and dispensaries where they're available—a direct feedback loop between marijuana producers and consumers that benefits both parties by rewarding the growers and retailers that provide the highest-quality experience. But it doesn't work in states where marijuana commerce remains underground.

For those still living behind the *irie* curtain, so to speak, simply finding something decent to smoke can be a chore, or far worse. Let's not forget, despite all the hoopla surrounding legalization, the land of the free continues to make more than 600,000 cannabis-related arrests every year, the vast majority for simple possession. So it's not exactly a buyer's market in Boise when it comes to things like finding your preferred Kush strain.

My advice to those left drooling from afar therefore would be to turn off the computer and invite a few humanoids over instead. Have each bring an eighth of the highest-quality weed they can acquire, then make up some scorecards, and host a small, private cannabis competition right in your own living room. Definitely create a fun prize for whoever supplies the top-rated strain, but don't let the stakes get too high, or take the contest aspect too seriously, lest the night end with sore feelings.

Instead, use the experience as an excuse to closely observe all that wonderful herb. Start by inhaling the scent of each offering when freshly ground and noting the subtle (or not so subtle) differences between them. Then take a "dry toke" off a joint prior to lighting it, or use a vaporizer, to get a pure taste of each strain before combustion turns it into smoke. And then, at last, you can start blazing, allowing ample time between sampling sessions to properly assess the effect—mental, physical, and emotional—of each strain, and how smoothly and evenly it burns, before moving on to the next.

Even as a veteran of more than twenty Cannabis Cups, both foreign and domestic, I still wouldn't call myself an expert, but thanks to rigorously following this process, I most definitely know "the best of the best" when I see, smell, taste, and inhale it. Though whenever anyone asks me my favorite strain, rather than start a debate, I invariably reply: "Whatever you've got!"

THE STRAIN IN SPAIN

Since 1983, author Jorge Cervantes has sold well over 1 million cop-ies of his acclaimed book *Marijuana Horticulture*, now published in seven languages. He's also a tireless researcher into the plant's many divergent genetic lines who constantly travels the globe visiting the planet's most skillful cannabis growers and sampling their goods.

So when *High Times* decided to produce a series of instructional marijuana cultivation DVDs, shot on location as Jorge explored the world's finest cannabis gardens, I jumped at the chance to direct.

Each DVD took weeks to shoot, during which time we typically visited two different growers per day, all of whom learned their lu-crative trade by reading Jorge's book. So needless to say, we had a warm welcome wherever we went, including a chance to sample myriad different marijuana varieties—occasionally with the men and women who bred them. In Spain, in particular, our little film crew had the unique pleasure of experiencing a foreign country and cul-ture from the inside. Welcomed into the better homes and gardens of growers from all walks of life, we shared ganja, wine, food, laughs, and as much language as we had in common. And everywhere we went, they grew the same strain: Jack Herer.

At the time, Spain was still in the early stages of its recent moves toward cannabis liberation, which meant most growers made due with whatever variety they could get their hands on. And Jack Herer was definitely the best of what was around. Named for a legendary cannabis activist and author, who wrote the seminal legalization manifesto *The Emperor Wears No Clothes*, the much-beloved Jack Herer cannabis variety is "the Champagne of strains," according to the exalted breeders at Sensi Seeds. It is also, truly, my favorite.

One afternoon, when we wrapped filming for the day, some

growers up in the Basque country invited Jorge, me, and the rest of our film crew to their private eating club for an unforgettable meal of local delicacies. When one of them proudly lit up a joint of locally grown Jack Herer between dinner and dessert, it suddenly occurred to me that my gracious hosts might not know the story behind the name. After all, Jack Herer, who passed away in 2010, remained a largely obscure figure even in his home country, despite helping to ignite America's modern marijuana revolution.

So I asked my new Basque friend, in my best attempt at stoned Spanish:

"¿Sabes Jack Herer no es solamente una planta, pero es un hombre también?"

["Do you know that Jack Herer is not only a plant, but also a man?"]

At which point, silence descended between us, as he took in what I'd said. And then replied: *"Jack Herer es un hombre magnífico, no?"*

POT SHOPPING

Whether you're buying recreational weed in Colorado, medical marijuana in Michigan, or ordering off a coffee-shop menu in Amsterdam, the retail cannabis experience remains both delightful and disorienting to the unaccustomed. So here's a few tips for keeping your wits about you when faced with all those wonderful choices.

Make a Budget for Getting Bud

Unless you grow your own, or have some lovely hookup, cannabis is most definitely a luxury item. So while it's certainly OK to splurge on the herb from time to time, that's a decision best made in advance, not once you're faced with a menu of enticing strains, concentrates, and edibles. Decide in advance how much you can afford to spend and how long it's got to last, and you'll have a lot of fun weighing your options when the time comes, without stressing out about next month's rent.

Look for Deals, Not Strains

Unless you're dead set on acquiring some hot new variety that everybody's talking about on your marijuana message boards, it's best to let the early adopters pay a premium for the latest craze and keep an eye out for hot deals instead. Retailers discount a product for all manner of reasons, and many also offer special coupons through their websites, so there's no reason to pay top dollar for an all-natural herb that already costs way too much.

Go Sun-Grown

That perfect little nugget in the dispensary display jar may look pristine, but it probably came from a warehouse-size factory farm–style indoor grow room with thousands of plants packed together in artificial, disposable growing mediums, under energy-intensive lights powered by fossil fuels, and fed chemical fertilizers that are used once then thrown away. At one time, such input-heavy indoor growing was an unfortunate necessity of surviving prohibition, but now it's time to move the herb back out into the sunlight. Something we can all play a role in by sourcing the most ethically produced, environmentally responsible pot possible.

"As a cannabis consumer, your purchases will directly affect how marijuana is commercially grown, so you have a unique opportunity to encourage and support proper cultivation practices," an eco-minded outdoor marijuana farmer from the organization Grow It in the Sun once informed me. "Cows should have the right to organic, sun-grown grass, and so should you."

The Smell Test

Your olfactory sense is incredibly refined when it comes to predicting what your body does (and doesn't) want to ingest, so if a bud or concentrate smells particularly alluring to you, go for it. For while cannabinoids like THC and CBD are odorless, the plant's terpenes (see pages 39–41) do provide an effective way to judge both potency and quality by smell. And conversely, definitely "turn up your nose" at any offering that smells funky, moldy, or like chemicals.

Never Buy a Pre-Roll

Every pre-rolled joint on Earth—from Amsterdam to Anchorage—is made by collecting the shake at the bottom of a giant bag of weed and grinding it up with the smallest, least-potent buds, all to make a product you then pay a premium for compared to buying the best buds of the same strain. So if you do know how to roll a joint, there's no excuse for being so lazy, and if you don't know how to roll, turn to page 60 immediately!

Never Hesitate to Investigate

If you're lucky enough to live in (or visit) a place with multiple cannabis retail options, don't ever settle for an establishment that makes you feel less than welcome, even if you've got a million annoying questions about every little thing. Because if they're not interested in helping you access the best possible information, odds are they're not interested in acquiring the best cannabis possible either, or serving as a positive example for the industry. So even if you've got to go a little farther to get there, find a marijuana retailer that makes you feel safe and accepted, including by answering all your queries with grace and patience.

ACCOUTREMENTS

Smoking pot properly requires precious little equipment. Personally, I've puffed out of a $25,000 blown-glass dinosaur that ranks among my favorite interactive art pieces of all time, and gotten just as high using a hollowed-out apple—that I later ate, lest it go to waste. So don't ever feel compelled to spend a lot of money on pot stuff, though there are a few essentials that you really can't live the high life without.

Grinder

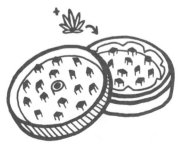

A thorough grinding properly prepares your herb for the flame by increasing its surface area, so it burns evenly. Resist the temptation to pick up a cheap plastic or poorly made metal grinder, as they quickly gunk up with resin and become permanently stuck. Instead, find a high-quality stainless steel grinder and clean it regularly with co- conut oil or isopropyl alcohol to ensure it lives as long as you do.

Rolling Papers

First of all, any kind of "flavored" rolling paper is definitely ketchup on a steak if you've got some nice, tasty bud to smoke. And even if you're stuck blaz- ing terrible weed (and we've all been there), you're still far better off just acquiring that taste and then chasing it with an actual straw- berry than you are inhaling some crazy artificial strawberry flavoring that's been sprayed onto your rollies.

Most gas stations and convenience stores carry a wide array of rolling papers in all sizes, so skip the dumb stuff and go for the ones made with raw, unbleached paper. (Hemp paper is also great, but a bit harder to roll.) As for blunts, that's your choice to smoke tobacco, but I don't mess with it.

Bat

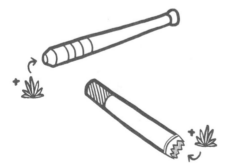

Back when I still lived in NYC, I took a bat with me everywhere. No, not to de- fend myself from ruffians, and not that kind of bat. I'm talking about a small metal (or ceramic) pipe made to look like a ciga- rette for public use. Designed for packing and puffing discreetly, the bat offered me a lot of peace of mind in a city where countless citizens get arrested every year for smoking weed (yes, me once included), so I highly recommend it for anyone interested in an occasional clandestine session while on the go.

Rolling Tray

You don't have to buy a "rolling tray"; just track down an existing tray and start rolling on it. Get creative, and you'll find a lot of interesting contenders already in your home. Or take the next step, and either buy or construct a "resin-catching" rolling tray with a fine mesh screen to roll on, and a glass slate underneath to capture all the trichomes that get dislodged from your bud and fall through the screen during the rolling process. These resin catchers collect a surprising amount of trichomes over time, which you can press into a kief-style hashish or sprinkle onto a joint for added potency.

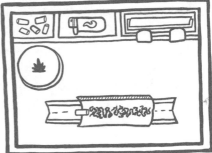

Pipe

No easier way to smoke weed than out of a pipe, which also makes fairly efficient use of your stash, provided you grind your herb thoroughly before packing it, and allow it to burn smoothly and evenly once lit. Glass tastes great and works beautifully if kept clean, but be wary of extremely cheap pipes sold in corner stores and some head shops, as they're imported from Asia and India, where their manufacturing process is poorly regulated.

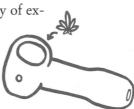

So make the investment in a locally

blown glass piece—even if it means spending a little more. You won't have to worry about strange chemicals or glass dust in your pipe, and you'll be supporting a true artisan in your home-grown cannabis community.

Vaporizer

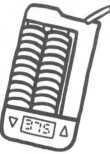

In 2015, the Wirecutter—a major consumer product review website—asked me to look at the fast-growing portable vaporizer market, do extensive testing, and then pick my favorite. At first, I was hesitant, because although I recognize the health benefits of vaporizing over smoking, I have to admit that I just didn't do it that often. (Though I'm sure I'd carry a vape pen if I still lived in New York, as a technological "upgrade" from smoking my old analog bat.)

Anyway, I'm glad I took the assignment, because people often ask me for a recommendation and now I can offer them some serious guidance. Like, definitely avoid any cheaply constructed product with plastic parts, or any vaporizer that emits a funny smell other than burning herb. Instead, look for something that's built to last, from appropriate materials. For more detailed advice, check out my Wirecutter article online, which will be updated regularly as new products come out.

Bong

A 2001 scientific study by the Multidisciplinary Association for Psychedelic Studies and California NORML found that using a water pipe to smoke marijuana actually filters out contaminants and cannabinoids in equal measure, rendering so-called bongs "ineffectual at improving the THC/tar ratio in cannabis smoke." Which means there's no real health benefit to them, and you're losing a lot of your stash to the filtering process, but still—*huge bong rips!*

In any event, if you do decide to own a bong, you must keep it squeaky clean, even if the rest of your home is an absolute shithole.

Mute

If you're still stuck smoking weed behind the *irie* curtain, kindly consider constructing a simple mute to eliminate those incriminating odors. Just stuff a paper-towel tube with (nontoxic!) dryer sheets, rubber band a paper towel or gas mask over one end, and exhale all of your hits into the other end. Warning, this is far from a foolproof system, especially if you're not diligent when using the mute. And extra especially if you have a bunch of people using it at once who aren't diligent. Still, like the rhythm method of birth control, it's way better than nothing.

Oil Rig

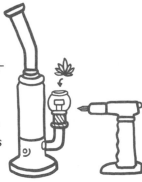

If you've ever thought getting high should involve a blowtorch and a glowing-hot titanium nail, these glass water pipes designed specifically for "dabbing" BHO cannabis concentrates will make you smile. Again, beware of cheap knockoffs with loose fittings, mouthpieces dangerously close to the nail, and light, frail glass walls.

EAT YOUR WEEDIES

In June 2014, I wrote an opinion piece for VICE titled "Maureen Dowd Freaked Out on Weed Chocolate Because She's Stupid." In it, I took the inexplicably popular *New York Times* columnist to task for her musings of a day earlier, in which she'd described enduring a total meltdown after going one bite over the line on a legal marijuana edible purchased in Colorado.

"Sitting in my hotel room in Denver, I nibbled off the end and then, when nothing happened, nibbled some more," Dowd wrote of her ill-fated journey. "For an hour, I felt nothing. . . . Then I felt a scary shudder go through my body and brain. I barely made it from the desk to the bed, where I lay curled up in a hallucinatory state for the next eight hours. . . . I was panting and paranoid, sure that when the room-service waiter knocked and I didn't answer, he'd call the police and have me arrested for being unable to handle my candy."

Naturally, I couldn't help but note that a veteran reporter, literally on assignment to investigate marijuana legalization, didn't consult the label or bother asking the trained, state-licensed employees she copped her cannabis "candy" from about the potency of the chocolate, how much THC a novice user should ingest, how long it would take to onset, how long the high would last, or what to do if she got too high. I also made it clear that I don't really think she's stupid, just that she acted stupidly in this instance—something even smart people do from time to time.

Which means that as long as there's cannabis-infused cupcakes on this Earth, somebody will always eat too much. Luckily, while 1,500 people die from accidental alcohol poisoning every year in America, nobody in human history has ever fatally overdosed on marijuana. So if you ever do go overboard on edibles, just remember that while you may feel like you're dying, you're not. An overly intense marijuana experience can be both psychologically alarming and physically debilitating, but it will pass in time without any lasting damage to your body or mind.

So try retreating to a quiet, dimly lit place and putting on soothing music or a familiar, funny movie to help you relax. Stay hydrated, talk with a trusted friend, and eat some non-infused food if possible, to slow the onset of the still-undigested THC in your stomach. Also, according to the Zendo Project, an onsite harm-reduction service providing compassionate care for individuals having difficult psychedelic experiences, it's important to avoid the "bad trip" mind-set in these instances. Instead, breathe deep, settle in, and try to use the experience as an opportunity for transcendence.

"Difficult psychedelic experiences can be frightening, but they are also potentially among the most valuable experiences someone can have," according to Zendo's official *Psychedelic Training Harm Reduction Manual*. "By working with these experiences . . . the psychedelic user can make [them] a chance for personal growth."

Or you could always go one better and avoid overdosing on edibles in the first place. That's been my approach ever since a parking-lot treat sent me spinning at a Grateful Dead show one fateful, youthful night back when ingesting ganja was just my passion, not my job. For many years after that frightening evening spent wandering Shakedown Street in a haze, you couldn't get me to eat a pot brownie even if you covered it with ice cream.

So how'd I go from avoiding edibles entirely to writing a column for VICE called The Weed Eater and producing a video series for them called *Bong Appetit*? Or more precisely, what convinced me to try digesting the herb again after a solid decade of sticking to smoking?

It was a trip to the magical chocolate factory in Oakland, California, where master chocolatier Scott Van Rixel produces his lovely Bhang bars. Already a successful entrepreneur with his own retail shop and national line of "normal" chocolate bars when he founded Bhang in 2010, Van Rixel was among the first wave of pedigreed businesspeople from the straight world who started entering the cannabis industry around that time. So I wrote a feature about him for *High Times* not long after he made the leap.

"We need to operate in a way that earns the respect of government officials, law enforcement, and the wider community," Van Rixel explained at the outset of my chocolate factory tour. "If they don't believe in what you're making, at least make them believe in how you're making it."

To that end, he concluded the tour by handing me a Bhang bar that, THC aside, looked ready for the shelves at Whole Foods, including childproof packaging and a label that met FDA standards for food and herbal supplement products—all at a time when even fully state-compliant medical-marijuana suppliers still faced a serious threat of federal raids. Under "other ingredients," Bhang's flagship dark chocolate bar—a vegan option with 73.5 percent premium, organic, fairly traded Venezuelan criollo cocoa—listed 60 milligrams of THC and less than 2 milligrams each of CBD and CBN. The bar was easily broken into four separate segments; each offering a single 15-milligram dose of edible THC.

Nowadays, Van Rixel no longer fears law enforcement, but his Bhang bars do face stiff competition from a wide range of equally appealing edibles. Still, he was surely the first to market with a product that combined high-quality ingredients and preparation, professional packaging and labeling, and verified lab-tested potency information. And so when I got that home that night, after a bit of hesitation, my wife and I each ate a 15-milligram segment—and it changed our lives. For the first time, we could enjoy the wonderful high of marijuana-infused food with a clear idea of how much THC we'd eaten. Which sounds like a simple thing, but imagine if every time someone handed you a glass of wine it varied so widely in potency that after drinking it you might end up feeling mildly buzzed or completely blotto, with no way to know which in advance.

Add in the fact that the effects of marijuana edibles can take up to ninety minutes to onset, and that absorbing THC through the liver when eaten (as opposed to through the lungs when smoked) actually converts it into a far stronger form of the drug, and you've got a recipe for potential disaster. Unless, unlike Ms. Dowd at the *Times*, you take the time to do a little research and ask a few questions before going back for that second bite.

For example, when Marinol, a synthetic form of THC sold as a prescription drug, was tested for FDA approval, researchers determined that for novice users, 2.5 milligrams was barely perceptible or imperceptible, 5 milligrams was clearly perceptible to most participants, and 10 milligrams was significantly noticeable to most recipients. Assuming you're already pretty comfortable with the effects of smoking pot, and want something ever so slightly stronger than "significantly noticeable," I'd say 15 milligrams is a good place to start. And don't go back for more until at least two hours after your initial dose—or try to drive while impaired on marijuana edibles, or do your taxes (at least without rechecking them later).

Incredible Edibles

Once we dialed in our preferred dosage of THC, my wife and I found ourselves turning to edibles more and more—as a healthier alternative to both smoking and alcohol; as a way to treat chronic pain, anxiety, and insomnia without pharmaceutical drugs; and as a special treat to share with friends at concerts, festivals, and dinner parties. Since we both love to cook, we quickly moved from store-bought chocolates and cookies to making our own cannabis-infused food at home.

Elise would go on to write *The Official High Times Cannabis Cookbook*, which *Vogue*'s Jeffrey Steingarten praised as "in a category of its own—intelligent, savvy, and knowledgeable about food, with excellent general information about cannabis and cooking with it." She's since been interviewed by the *New York Times*, *Los Angeles Times*, *Bon Appétit*, and dozens of other major publications and media outlets, and traveled the world educating people about how to safely prepare and enjoy marijuana-infused food.

Elise also serves as head of judging in the edibles category for the *High Times* Cannabis Cup as it tours the world every year, which means we've both been keeping well up to date on the latest offerings from the fastest-growing segment of America's legal cannabis industry. So when VICE's food channel, Munchies, contacted me about contributing a monthly column on cannabis and cuisine, I felt as well prepared as anyone (except perhaps my own wife) to take a deep look at the way these two worlds intersect.

In the first installment, I tried to set the tone properly.

Brace yourself, because together we're about to embark on a cannabis-fueled culinary journey. . . . Like adventurers following the spice roads of old, we'll traverse an ancient, storied, and sometimes perilous route rife with exotic ingredients, bold flavors, and colorful characters—quite naturally stopping to sample the goods all along the way—wherever high-end cuisine intersects with getting high.

Never did this quest reach a higher peak than in Aspen, where I hosted a special video installment of The Weed Eater, featuring a five-course cannabis-infused gourmet dinner prepared by one of the city's top chefs, and served at Owl Farm—the former home and fortified compound of Hunter S. Thompson. On so many levels, the entire experience was a dream come true, starting with the raison d'être for this celebration, namely the legalization of marijuana in Colorado. Also, I'm a huge Hunter Thompson fan (we even share the same birthday).

Most people know that the late, great Gonzo legend behind *Fear and Loathing in Las Vegas* and some of the twentieth century's funniest and most insightful journalism enjoyed marijuana (among other things) immensely, but his tireless activism in pushing for the herb's legalization on the grounds of limited government and personal liberty has been less well documented. So with the kind permission of his widow, Anita, who resides at Owl Farm and keeps a close eye on her dearly departed husband's literary legacy, we threw a victory dinner in honor of Thompson's cannabis colleague and close friend Keith Stroup, founder of the National Organization for the Reform of Marijuana Laws (NORML)—America's oldest and largest organization promoting pot legalization.

Keith and Hunter met for the first time at the 1972 Democratic National Convention, and quickly formed a bond based on more than shared politics, as Keith explains in the Munchies video:

> *NORML was only about a year and a half old, and the first day I was at the convention, I clearly smelled marijuana smoke coming up from under the bleachers where I was sitting. So I looked down, and I saw this gangling figure down there. We'd never met, but I'd seen pictures of him in* Rolling Stone, *and I thought,*

*"Son of a bitch, that has to be Hunter Thompson." So I went
down there, introduced myself, and said, "I just started a marijuana lobby called NORML, maybe we should get to know
each other."*

*And, of course, he held out the joint to me and said, "You
want some?" and we formed a friendship that lasted till his
death.*

To tackle the culinary feat of preparing a multicourse
marijuana-infused meal of the highest order, I partnered chef
Chris Lanter of Aspen hotspot Cache Cache with Denver-based
cannabis-infusion expert Tamar Wise, former head of science at
Dixie Botanicals, the world's largest marijuana edibles company.
Together, they infused four different oils, using four different
ganja strains, for use in four different preparations (three savory
and one dessert). Tamar normally works with industrial-grade
equipment designed to make large-scale infusions for use in
commercial products, but on this occasion, she agreed to put
her multiple advanced degrees and years of hands-on experience
to work in formulating a simple but highly efficient and accurate infusion procedure for home cooks.

Without a doubt, this is definitely the method you should
use when making cannabis-infused food at home. Other
methods "work," of course, but not as accurately or efficiently. Which is why I call Tamar's method "How to Make
Marijuana-Infused Food (Without Wasting Weed or Freaking
Out!)."

HOW TO MAKE MARIJUANA-INFUSED FOOD (WITHOUT WASTING WEED OR FREAKING OUT!)

STEP 1: DETERMINING PROPER DOSAGE

Start by determining the potency of the cannabis you're working with, always using a high estimate to avoid overdosing. For smoking-grade buds, use 15 percent THC (20 percent for super kind), and use 10 percent for high-quality "trim." Then determine your cannabis's total amount of THC by weighing it in grams. (One gram of 20 percent THC bud contains 200 total milligrams of THC.)

In raw, dried cannabis, the plant's THC largely exists in a non-psychoactive acidic form that must be heated to the point of decarboxylation in order to convert this THC-A into psychoactive THC. Most "pot brownie" recipes call for doing this while making the infusion, but it's far more efficient to decarb your pot first in the oven and then infuse it into butter or oil on the stove top—a two-step method that also keeps the integrity of both the oil and the cannabis more intact.

To accurately estimate the THC concentration of your finished infusion, first start by determining the total amount of THC in your starting material (as described above). Then estimate extraction efficiency at 80 percent. And finally, measure exactly how much butter or oil you will infuse your cannabis into, in order to figure out an estimated dose per teaspoon once infused.

For example:

If you infuse one stick of butter (24 teaspoons) with 1 gram of cannabis, that's 20 percent THC (200 total milligrams) and achieve an 80 percent extraction efficiency, you'll yield

*an infusion with approximately 160 milligrams of psycho-
active THC (or 6.66 milligrams per teaspoon, which is actually a really good target to shoot for, dosage-wise).*

STEP 2: MAKING THE INFUSION

Preheat the oven to 240 degrees F.

Grind cannabis sufficiently to increase surface area without turning it into powder, then spread it evenly on the bottom of a hotel pan or baking sheet. Place it in the middle of the oven and allow the cannabis to decarboxylate for 1 hour and 15 minutes, stirring halfway through. Then remove it from the oven and let cool for 10 minutes.

Meanwhile, fill a small spray bottle with grain alcohol (Everclear) and spray a light, fine mist of it over the ground cannabis. Stir with a spoon and lightly spray again. This will help break down the plant's cellulose, allowing for a more efficient THC infusion with less green color. (If you don't have a spray bottle, you can use a teaspoon and sprinkle the Everclear on while stirring.) Let cannabis sit after the Everclear step for 15 minutes. Then bring oil or butter up to temperature slowly. Since we have already decarboxylated the cannabis, the oil needs to be hot enough only to extract cannabinoids (not decarb them). Bring to a very slow simmer and then spoon cannabis into it while stirring gently.

Keep on a slow simmer for at least 30 minutes, and ideally 6 hours for maximum efficiency, stirring occasionally and never letting it reach a boiling point. Once infusion is done, turn off the heat and let the infusion cool for at least 20 minutes. While the infusion cools, line a strainer with cheesecloth. Pour the infusion through the cheesecloth to separate out plant matter. Strain more than once if needed.

The infusion is now ready to use. The easiest way to use these infusions is by simply drizzling them on food immediately before serving, keeping track of the dosage by measuring it out one teaspoon at a time. Always label marijuana-infused food clearly, and keep it away from children, animals, and anyone who might unknowingly ingest it. Refrigerate when not in use (in a clearly marked container not accessible to children!). Will keep for about 2 weeks.

YOU'RE DOING A HECK OF A JOB, BROWNIE

Cannabis legalization has led to incredible advances in the quality and variety of store-bought marijuana edibles on the market, at least for those lucky enough to live in a place with retail sales. I've personally sampled THC-infused macaroons, biscotti, beef jerky, ice cream, and bonbons that can more than hold their own against the world's best "straight" food. And yet nothing will ever displace society's deeply ingrained reverence for the humble "pot brownie," which is so hardwired into our cultural DNA that it's pretty much become the de facto platonic ideal of marijuana-laced treats. But have you ever wondered why?

While gooey, rich chocolatey brownies undoubtedly do an excellent job of masking and thus making palatable the "grassy" taste of cannabis, the real history of the pot brownie derives not from a winning flavor combination but from a high-profile prank among the intelligentsia.

Once a leading light of Parisian literary society, author and critic Gertrude Stein left her home, estate, and extensive art collection to her longtime romantic partner Alice B. Toklas when she died in 1946, but Toklas later lost everything in court when French authorities refused to recognize the legitimacy of the couple's committed relationship. So in an effort to raise funds, Toklas tried to get by with a little help from her friends by having them help her assemble a bohemian cookbook. Which inspired a painter named Brion Gysin to have a little fun by submitting a recipe for Haschich [*sic*] Fudge.

Toklas, who had little to no experience with hashish, missed the joke, and included the recipe without understanding its potency, though Gysin's strange introductory text (not to mention the "bunch of canibus [*sic*]" listed among the ingredients) probably should have tipped her off.

"This is the food of paradise—of Baudelaire's Artificial Paradises," the recipe promised, referencing the famed Club des Hashischins. "Euphoria and brilliant storms of laughter; ecstatic reveries and extensions of one's personality on several simultaneous planes are to be complacently expected."

The fudge's inclusion in *The Alice B. Toklas Cook Book* would eventually lead to international controversy (and plenty of extra book sales). The first American edition omitted the recipe, but a later version published it in time to become a go-to guide for countless beatniks and hippies looking to get high— even though, as anyone who actually attempted to make Haschich Fudge quickly discovered, the actual Alice B. Toklas recipe doesn't much resemble fudge (or a brownie), as it has no chocolate, and is completely raw.

By the time pop culture jumped into the mix, however, with the delightful 1968 Peter Sellers movie *I Love You, Alice B. Toklas*, that complex concoction (replete with dates, figs, almonds, nutmeg, black peppercorn, cinnamon, coriander, butter, and sugar) was replaced on-screen with a box of brownie mix and a handful of weed. And from then on, it was just pot brownies all the way down. . . .

If you want to try the original recipe, look for it online, or better yet pick up a copy of *The Alice B. Toklas Cook Book*, and in the meantime here's my favorite recipe for a classic pot brownie that's delicious and easy to make.

—— CLASSIC POT BROWNIE RECIPE ——

INGREDIENTS

1 cup all-purpose flour
¼ cup unsweetened cocoa powder
½ teaspoon salt
½ teaspoon baking powder
3 tablespoons cannabis-infused oil
5 ounces semisweet chocolate, chopped
1 cup firmly packed light brown sugar
½ tablespoon light corn syrup
1 tablespoon applesauce
3 egg whites
2 teaspoons vanilla

1. Preheat oven to 350°F.
2. Mix together flour, cocoa powder, salt, and baking powder in a small bowl and set aside.
3. Pour the cannabis-infused oil and chopped chocolate into a double boiler over high heat. As water boils in the lower pan, whisk oil and chocolate until melted and smooth. Remove from heat, and whisk in brown sugar, corn syrup, and applesauce. Stir in egg whites and vanilla. Beat mixture vigorously until smooth, then stir in flour mixture until fully incorporated.
4. Grease a 9-by-13-inch baking pan. Pour batter into pan. Bake for approximately 20 minutes, or until the center of the top is almost firm to touch. Let cool. Enjoy responsibly! Stones 16.

NONNA MARIJUANA'S
CHICKEN POT-CHIATORI

I know ninety-three-year-old Aurora Leveroni as the woman who birthed and raised my friend Valerie Corral (cofounder of WAMM, California's oldest and most compassionate medical-cannabis collective). But the world now knows Aurora best as kindhearted, wisecracking Nonna Marijuana, after she stole the show (and went viral) in the first-ever installment of *Bong Appetit*.

In the episode, we meet Nonna, learn how she's been home-cooking amazing Italian food for more than eighty years, and then take a guided tour of WAMM's extensive medicinal garden before heading into the kitchen to prepare an amazing cannabis-infused feast.

Nothing I write here can possibly do justice to just how funny and warm Nonna is (in the video, and in real life), so just head over to YouTube and check out the episode next time you need a laugh or a surrogate grandma. In the meantime, here's Nonna's recipe for her signature dish.

Bong Appetit!

NONNA MARIJUANA'S
CHICKEN POT-CHIATORI

INGREDIENTS

1 fryer chicken, cut into pieces (leave skin on)
Salt and pepper, to taste
3 tablespoons cannabis-infused butter
1 tablespoon olive oil
1 large onion, cut into thumb-size pieces

¼ cup small cremini mushrooms
About ½ glass of white wine (optional)
¼ cup black olives with pits
¼ cup Sicilian plain olives (no pits)
¼ cup green olives with pits
¼ cup green olives stuffed with garlic or pimento

1. Wash and dry the chicken and sprinkle with salt and pepper.
2. Slowly heat the weed-infused butter and olive oil in a skillet, then add the fryer pieces until well-browned.
3. Remove the pieces and place onto a plate.
4. Using the same pan you used to fry the chicken, lower the heat and fry the onion pieces until transparent. Replace the chicken pieces and add the cremini mushrooms, continuing to cook on low heat for about 5 minutes.
5. Add the white wine and let it sizzle. Now, add all the olives, gently stirring to combine. Cover until ready to serve.

ELEVATED GOO-BALLS

Most of the prepackaged edibles available at legal marijuana stores and medical-marijuana dispensaries fall somewhere between gummy bears and snickerdoodles when it comes to nutritional value. So they're basically taking one of the healthiest foods you can put into your body, cannabis, and cutting it with a heavy dose of a dangerous, highly addictive drug called sugar.

Fortunately, some of the larger edibles manufacturers have started to offer at least one healthy choice, and a growing number of boutique specialty operations have sprouted up to cater to those seeking sugar-free, gluten-free, vegan, paleo, and even raw options, but that's still the vast exception to the rule, and only for those with access to a large, well-stocked retail cannabis outlet. So my wife decided to "elevate" the traditional Grateful Dead parking lot goo-ball into a true superfood, featuring both the nutritional boost of hemp seeds and the medicinal/spiritual high of cannabis resin. They're great for munching on long hikes or before a concert. And because she carefully measures dosage to ensure each ball's around 10 milligrams THC, I never have to worry about missing the second set with a massive case of the bummers.

AMAZEBALLS

DRY INGREDIENTS

1 cup unsalted raw almonds, coarsely chopped
½ cup shredded coconut
½ cup raisins
½ cup rolled oats
¼ cup pumpkin seeds
¼ cup hulled hemp seeds
¼ cup sunflower seeds
2 tablespoons cacao powder
1 tablespoon flax powder or other superfood booster, such as maca, spirulina, or hemp protein (optional)

WET INGREDIENTS

8 large Medjool dates (about 1 cup)
½ cup Canna-Coconut Oil, melted (recipe follows)
⅓ cup almond butter
¼ cup sunflower seed butter
1 tablespoon agave nectar
1 tablespoon hemp oil

FOR COATING THE BALLS

⅓ cup shredded coconut
⅓ cup hulled hemp seeds

1. Place the chopped almonds in a large bowl, add all remaining dry ingredients, and mix thoroughly.
2. Place all wet ingredients into the bowl of a food processor, and blend until completely combined.
3. Use a spoon to mix wet ingredients into dry ingredients.
4. Put a layer of shredded coconut on a plate and a layer of hemp seeds on another plate. Form mixture into balls (about 2 inches in diameter) with your hands, so each ball is just big enough for one or two bites. Roll balls into hemp seed, then roll in coconut to coat surface entirely. Place the finished balls into an airtight container and refrigerate for at least 30 minutes to solidify. Eat with a nice cup of hot tea and enjoy! Makes 12 to 16 balls, and each ball is one daytime dose.

CANNA-COCONUT OIL

INGREDIENTS

1 ounce cannabis, dried, or 2 ounces trimmed leaf
1 (14-ounce) jar coconut oil

1. Fill a pot halfway with water, and add cannabis. Bring to a simmer, stirring occasionally for 1 hour.
2. Add coconut oil, and return to a simmer.
3. Remove from heat. Let coconut oil mixture sit in a covered pot for 2 days as it slowly extracts.
4. Reheat mixture over medium-low heat until oil melts. Strain mixture into a bowl, being sure to press plant matter firmly

against the side of the strainer. Refrigerate the mixture, covered, for at least 24 hours.

5. Return the next day and, using a butter knife, separate solidified oil from water. Pat the solidified canna-coconut oil dry
with a paper towel and then melt in a saucepan until it is liquid.
Then pour measured amounts into glass jars for easy dosing.

HOW TO SMOKE POT (MEDICINALLY)

Dr. Jeffrey Hergenrather, head of the Society of Cannabis Clini-
cians, first learned of marijuana's incredible therapeutic value
more than forty years ago, while serving as house doctor at the
Farm—a legendary counterculture commune that was founded
in rural Tennessee in 1971 and is still operational today.

Since he had such a large patient base in those days (more than
1,000 residents at the height of the Farm), and pretty much all
those patients felt comfortable confiding in their long-haired,
joint-smoking doc about their own pot use, Hergenrather became
one of the first MDs of the modern era to get a true sense of just
how many seemingly unrelated ailments cannabis can effectively
treat—without the side effects, addiction, and secondary health
problems so often associated with pharmaceutical drugs.

Unfortunately, nowadays, while medical cannabis is increasingly accepted, and study after study suggests marijuana is a
true "miracle drug," Dr. Hergenrather says too many otherwise
competent physicians still don't know the truth about this healing herb.

"For the most part, my generation of doctors has no idea
what's going on," he told me in a 2011 *High Times* interview.
"There was no recognition of the endocannabinoid system until

the mid-'90s, and they didn't start teaching it in medical school for another decade, so many physicians just don't understand that cannabinoids found in the marijuana plant activate and modulate an important natural system in the body in a way that logically accounts for all the varied benefits people claim to get from ingesting cannabis. Otherwise, it just doesn't sound right when you start talking about all the great things marijuana can do to help heal people. It's so unbelievable, many doctors just kind of say: 'No, thanks—I don't want to get involved.'"

Despite this deplorable level of ignorance, don't ever be afraid to talk openly and honestly with your physician about medical marijuana as an option, just do so without admitting to breaking the law, and be prepared to be the one providing an education on the subject. Someday, I'd like to write an entire book called *What Your Doctor Doesn't Know (Or Won't Tell You) About Medical Marijuana*, but for now, let's just focus on learning a few of the most important medicinal uses of the plant, relying on the most credible and accredited sources possible.

Cancer

Everybody knows that smoking a joint can work wonders for treating the severe nausea and pain associated with cancer and chemotherapy treatments, but lately there's been even more excitement around the idea that cannabis's chemical components can actually prevent cancer from forming, halt its progression, and even kill off existing cancerous cells.

All the way back in 1974, researchers sponsored by the National Institutes of Health published a paper in *The Journal of the National Cancer Institute* titled "Anticancer Activity of Cannabinoids" showing that compounds in marijuana were capable of shrinking tumors, but instead of following up on these findings, the government acted to effectively subvert all research into cannabis unless specifically designed to prove its harms.

Now, however, as a series of international follow-up studies have again proven cannabis's anti-tumor properties, and countless patients have come forward with dramatic tales of fighting advanced cancer successfully with highly concentrated cannabis oil, the US government has finally begun to back studies into how cannabinoids can be best utilized in treating the disease.

According to the American Cancer Society, "scientists [have] reported that THC and other cannabinoids such as CBD slow growth and/or cause death in certain types of cancer cells growing in laboratory dishes. . . . Some animal studies also suggest certain cannabinoids may slow growth and reduce spread of some forms of cancer."

Crohn's Disease/Inflammatory Bowel Disease

While the Crohn's and Colitis Foundation of America (CCFA) does not endorse the smoking of marijuana, any current state-based medical-marijuana programs, or the legalization of marijuana, their most recent position statement on medical marijuana (in 2012) did acknowledge experimental evidence that suggests "endocannabinoids, molecules found in the body that closely resemble compounds found in the cannabis (marijuana) plant, may play a role in limiting intestinal inflammation. Several small studies have shown that a significant proportion of patients with Inflammatory Bowel Disease (IBD) report smoking marijuana to relieve IBD-related symptoms, particularly those patients with a history of abdominal surgery, chronic abdominal pain, and/or a low quality of life index."

Recent studies at the Meir Medical Center in Israel further suggest cannabis to be a strong treatment option for controlling inflammation, abdominal pain, and other symptoms of inflammatory bowel disease, making cannabis a good alternative to steroid treatment, with benefits including improved appetite and sleep, with no significant side effects.

Epilepsy

Medical cannabis patients have known the profound effect cannabis can have on epilepsy and other seizure disorders for decades, but it wasn't until CNN's Dr. Sanjay Gupta reported on the way highly concentrated cannabis oil rich in CBD (a non-psychoactive cannabinoid) can potentially transform otherwise treatment-resistant pediatric epilepsy cases that the issue broke wide open. After all, when a child goes from hundreds of seizures every week to just a few per month, and that seizure reduction begins almost immediately upon her very first dose of cannabis oil, it's sort of hard to keep arguing that marijuana has no medicinal value.

In fact, laboratory research has already confirmed that CBD has demonstrated effectiveness at reducing seizure severity and producing anticonvulsant effects (University of Reading, 2010). Results also suggest that CBD could function well if co-prescribed with current treatment options to decrease dosages and their undesirable side effects (Virginia Commonwealth University, 2003). All of which prompted the US government in 2014 to begin quietly backing research into CBD as a potential pediatric epilepsy treatment through its investigational new drug program, as chronicled in a VICE story I wrote titled "The US Government Now Supplies Cannabis Extracts to Epileptic Kids."

Chronic Pain

When medical marijuana first became widely available in California, detractors frequently used to scoff at how "anybody can get a doctor's recommendation" by simply claiming lower back pain, as if that in any way changes marijuana's effectiveness as a medicine, or isn't the exact same way millions of people end up with prescriptions for pharmaceutical painkillers every year.

A 2008 study in *The Journal of the American Medical Association*, in fact, showed that Americans spend more than $86 billion a year treating back and neck pain, often with dangerous pills, and frequently with little improvement and serious side effects. While a slew of other studies have confirmed marijuana's efficacy for treating both debilitating chronic pain and less severe cases, with a comprehensive 2011 review in the *British Journal of Clinical Pharmacology* concluding it is "reasonable to consider cannabinoids as a treatment option for the management of chronic neuropathic pain with evidence of efficacy in other types of chronic pain such as fibromyalgia and rheumatoid arthritis as well."

HIV/AIDS

When the AIDS crisis began devastating the homosexual community in San Francisco in the early 1980s, it didn't take long for the many pot smokers among those afflicted to realize that marijuana provided unparalleled relief from the syndrome's most debilitating symptoms, including severe nausea and loss of appetite. As word spread, so did demand for safe access to the medicine, which led to the formation of unlicensed "buyer's clubs" and also the beginning of a serious push for legal protection for the seriously ill that would culminate in statewide ballot initiative Proposition 215, which made California the first state to allow medical marijuana.

More recently, a 2014 analysis published by a team of researchers at Louisiana State University in the journal *AIDS Research and Human Retroviruses* offered evidence that beyond symptom control, daily intake of cannabis can help slow down or potentially even reverse progression of HIV. And a 2003 study by Stanford University School of Medicine credited cannabis with also treating anxiety and depression in patients, a "side effect" that can greatly improve treatment outcomes.

Multiple Sclerosis

In 1997, Dr. Geoffrey Guy decided to "pop in" on a half-day symposium on the therapeutic uses of cannabis, organized by the MS Society (UK). He left the emotionally charged meeting deeply moved by the MS patients' accounts of how cannabis (then available only on the black market) greatly improved their quality of life. He also smelled a lucrative business opportunity.

Guy would go on to found GW Pharmaceuticals, a company licensed by the British government to cultivate cannabis for use in making "whole-plant extracts" with specific ratios of THC and CBD for use as prescription medicines. Sativex, a 1:1 blend administered as a sublingual spray, has been available since 2006 in Canada as a treatment for spasticity related to multiple sclerosis.

While not yet available in the United States, Sativex has since been approved for MS in eleven other countries (and counting) because cannabinoids are a proven and safe treatment for the condition. When it comes to administering this plant medicinally, however, always remember that whole-plant herbal marijuana remains the "gold standard," because smoking or vaporizing cannabis buds offers far faster onset and easier titration than a sublingual spray (or any other pharmaceutical application), at a much lower cost to patients, while providing a far wider array of active components.

Anxiety

A 2011 study at the University of São Paulo on subjects with social anxiety disorder found that CBD inhibited their fear of speaking in public, a main symptom of the condition. When dosed with CBD (rather than a placebo) prior to giving a public speech, test subjects exhibited "significantly reduced anxiety, cognitive impairment, and discomfort in their speech performance and significantly decreased alert [*sic*] in their anticipatory speech."

Which may come as a surprise to anyone who's had the exact opposite reaction to marijuana, namely experiencing something from minor discomfort to a full-blown panic attack after one too many bong rips. But such an increase in anxiety is invariably a negative reaction to THC, so if anxiety's your issue, try medicating with either CBD-rich cannabis or, better yet, a tincture, capsule, or edible with a ratio of CBD to THC (12:1 or more) that will provide therapeutic benefits without any mental discomfort.

🌿 PRO TIP 🌿

HERB IS THE HEALING

OF THE NATIONS

"It doesn't have a high potential for abuse, and there are very legitimate medical applications. In fact, sometimes marijuana is the only thing that works."

—DR. SANJAY GUPTA, "WHY I CHANGED
MY MIND ON WEED"

> "The biggest killer on the planet is stress, and I still think the best medicine is and always has been cannabis."
> —WILLIE NELSON

> "I used marijuana every day during chemotherapy. It gave me an appetite so I was able to eat and keep my strength up. It also helped with depression, and eased gastrointestinal pain. I have been a medicinal marijuana smoker for nine years now. . . . I also enjoy it before I watch *Game of Thrones*."
> —MELISSA ETHERIDGE, "POT GOT ME THROUGH"

Parkinson's/Alzheimer's/Stroke

A 2014 study by researchers at Tel Aviv University, and published in the journal *Clinical Neuropharmacology*, found that smoking whole-plant cannabis provided symptomatic relief in patients with Parkinson's disease, and resulted in "significant improvement after treatment in tremor, rigidity, and bradykinesia [slowness of movement]. There was also significant improvement of sleep and pain scores. No significant adverse effects of the drug were observed."

Israel has been a hotbed of cannabis research since creating a national medical-marijuana program in 2007. Scientists there are able to collect data based on a wide patient base using "whole-plant" cannabis (that is, buds), whereas the majority of cannabinoid research involves only single compounds.

Meanwhile, in the United States, vital research is still being obstructed by the very same federal government that holds Patent #6630507 ("Cannabinoids as neuroprotectants and antioxidants"), which states flatly that compounds found in cannabis are "useful in the treatment and prophylaxis of a wide variety of oxidation associated diseases, such as ischemic, age-related, inflammatory and autoimmune diseases . . . and are found to have particular application as neuroprotectants, for example in limiting neurological damage following . . . stroke and trauma, or in the treatment of neurodegenerative diseases, such as Alzheimer's disease, Parkinson's disease and HIV dementia."

PTSD

At least twenty-two US military veterans commit suicide every day, many of them suffering with post-traumatic stress disorder (PTSD). In treating this epidemic among our returning soldiers (and others from all walks of life who've suffered a traumatic incident), "modern medicine" largely relies on a cadre of pills that don't really treat the underlying condition, but do come with a host of terrible side effects, including addiction, antisocial behavior, and fatal overdoses.

Rates of prescription for these pharmaceuticals have nonetheless skyrocketed in the last decade (along with Big Pharma profits), while the US government has continued to block vital research into cannabis as a safer and more effective alternative.

Meanwhile, growing evidence from around the world shows cannabis can safely and effectively treat PTSD, including a 2014 study at the University of Haifa that showed "administering synthetic marijuana (cannabinoids) soon after a traumatic event can prevent PTSD-like symptoms in rats, caused by the trauma and by trauma reminders."

Insomnia

With Americans spending more than $33 billion per year on sleep aids of one kind or another, including many pills with serious side effects and addictive properties, it's important to know there's an all-natural, nontoxic herbal remedy that's proven to work. Those in need of a safer, better Ambien should seek cannabis medicine rich in CBD, or even better, if available, a nutraceutical-type capsule of CBN, an oxidation product of THC that's only about 10 percent as psychoactive as its antecedent, with a strongly sedative effect.

Otherwise, look for heavily *indica*-dominant varieties, as even THC in lower doses is known to aid sleep (while higher doses can sometimes have the opposite effect).

Diabetes

According to a 2013 study in *The American Journal of Medicine*, marijuana may help users stay trim and enjoy a lowered risk of developing diabetes, findings that confirmed earlier research that showed cannabinoids can positively affect blood sugar and help the body process caloric intake.

"The most important finding is that current users of marijuana appeared to have better carbohydrate metabolism than nonusers," according to Murray Mittleman, an associate professor of medicine at Harvard Medical School and the study's lead author. "Their fasting insulin levels were lower, and they appeared to be less resistant to the insulin produced by their body to maintain a normal blood-sugar level."

These findings may clash with our cultural conception of whacked-out stoners with the munchies binging on sugary sweets, but for those with diabetes or an increased risk of developing the disease, there's ample reason to believe that focusing on a healthy diet, regular exercise, *and* smoking weed in moderation will yield the best results. In fact, that's an excellent health regimen for pretty much everyone to follow.

ADDITIONAL CONDITIONS TREATABLE WITH CANNABIS INCLUDE, BUT ARE NOT LIMITED TO

ADD/ADHD, ALS, anorexia, arthritis, Asperger syndrome, asthma, autism, Bell's palsy, bulimia, depression, fibromyalgia, glaucoma, hepatitis C, hypertension, lupus, Lyme disease, migraines, neuropathy, PMS, psoriasis, and traumatic brain injury.

FROM CONNOISSEUR TO AFICIONADO

Now that we've completed our initial overview of the cannabis plant, including learning its history, botany, chemistry, and cultivation—plus how to smoke, vape, dab, and eat it (for fun, as medicine, or both)—let's pause for just a moment before moving on to the world of marijuana etiquette, to make a vital distinction between the two types of pot enthusiasts.

Dr. Lester Grinspoon, author of *Marihuana Reconsidered* (see page 160), once told me in an interview that his world-renowned best bud Carl Sagan didn't really give much thought to different strains of marijuana but did "enjoy the best of the best when made available." Which means the planet's most famous modern astronomer was not a cannabis *connoisseur*, defined as "an expert judge in matters of taste," but rather an *aficionado*, or "one who is very knowledgeable and passionate about a pastime."

I believe that's a vital distinction to make at this point in the book. For while it's certainly nice to have a pot palate so well developed you can tell the difference between Lemon Haze and Lemon Kush on the first puff, it does sort of risk missing the forest for the trees.

Remember, to go beyond legalization, into a bold, new, bright green future, we needn't convince our fellow citizens that cannabis smells great and gets you nicely toasted. Only that it saves lives, creates jobs, and makes communities safer—a sacred mission that requires first learning everything you can about this wonderful herb, and then planting those seeds of knowledge everywhere you go.

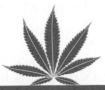

CHAPTER 3

Headiquette Lesson

Pass the Dutchie on the left-hand side,
don't Bogart that joint, and other
established customs of high society

When we talk about the rituals, ceremonies, and informal rules of etiquette that unite pot smokers, first and foremost comes an unwavering understanding that, in the immortal words widely attributed to American patriot Benjamin Franklin, "We must, indeed, all hang together, or most assuredly we shall all hang separately."

Which in turn brings to mind the time Jeff Dowd—real-life inspiration for the doobie-smoking detective known as "The Dude" in the classic Coen brothers film *The Big Lebowski*—waxed philosophic to me during a *High Times* interview about a seemingly fallow time in his life. A period he described as one of "heavy hanging."

So I asked if there's an art to hanging.

"Yeah, there's an art to hanging," the Dude replied. "And it starts with who you're hanging with."

Amen to that.

Without a doubt, there's been no greater pleasure in my time as a marijuana reporter than the incredible array of fascinating, kindhearted people—from all walks of life, across every demographic of race, age, religion, gender, sexual orientation, national origin, and political belief—that I've had the honor to hang heavy with and get to know over a few bowls. And the good news is that we're all part of one of the most inclusive, accessible subcultures you're ever likely to encounter. Even in the face of society's unfettered scorn and the surveillance state's unending paranoia campaign against us, the cannabis community remains open, welcoming, peaceful, and tolerant. Just discreetly greet any fellow member, say "high," and feel the love!

Nobody knows how to make new friends (and make the best of what's around) better than stoners. Then add in the fact that marijuana is not just a hobby or even a passion but also a social-justice movement, a cutting-edge medicine, and a rapidly emerging trillion-dollar global industry—and you're going to meet some interesting heads pretty much wherever and whenever you decide to get high. So when it comes to your private stash, share and share alike. And as for the rules of headiquette, definitely don't sweat the small stuff. Because any stoner circle that makes you feel bad about having the wrong rolling papers, or coughing too much, or passing a joint incorrectly, is actually the wrong stoner circle.

Authentic cannabis culture has been pushed so far underground for so long that nothing matters to real heads but your good name and your true self. Our customs are based on solidarity rather than exclusion, so instead of a litany of arbitrary rules to follow and elaborate costumes to wear, there's only four simple points of decorum to keep in mind.

Doob unto Others

Most marijuana etiquette stems from the good old Golden Rule ("Do unto others as you would have them do unto you"), plus a heady blend of common sense and good manners, with a little hashish sprinkled on top. So don't be an asshole, don't mooch herb all the time, don't come off high and mighty, and you'll be fine. (Please note that any action that makes you an asshole sans weed still makes you an asshole when stoned; it's not like drinking culture, where the inebriated get a free pass on some seriously horrific behavior.)

Most important, I can't tell you how many completely peaceful people I know who've had their doors busted down by armed authorities over relatively small amounts of herb, so even in our bold, new post-prohibition world, the one true prime directive when it comes to pot remains: *Don't get busted or get anybody else busted.*

Don't Smoke Weed with People You Don't Trust

One thing you may notice as your body's cannabinoid receptors become increasingly well lubricated is that while marijuana typically makes you more open and receptive to new people and ideas, you'll occasionally find yourself strongly repelled by someone—even if others react differently. Learn to trust these instincts. For just as ganja allows us to see ourselves more clearly, including our own bullshit, it also allows us to better detect the bullshit of others. Which explains why such a large majority of politicians oppose legalization, even though more than half the country is in favor.

Keep Your Head Held High

Like all oppressed minority groups, marijuana users have faced scapegoating, scare tactics, and false stereotypes meant to demonize and demean us. So now that the squares and the establishment at long last seem ready to rethink cannabis culture's place in polite society, how can we represent ourselves proudly and properly in the wider world—without forgetting our roots, or losing our cool?

"We're weeding out the stoners," advertising executive Olivia Mannix recently told the *New York Times* in a story about how a new breed of entrepreneur wants to change marijuana's image by framing it as a standard consumer product, like Coca-Cola or McDonald's, rather than a lifestyle choice or political cause. "We want to show the world that normal, professional, successful people consume cannabis."

Which means she must see frequent pot smokers as abnormal, unprofessional failures. Or, more charitably, she believes the world sees "stoners" that way after a century of government propaganda, and that image is getting in the way of her clients making money. Either way, while Ms. Mannix and I agree that the public's perception of marijuana consumers is a problem facing not just the cannabis industry but the culture at large, I have a far different solution. Instead of telling people that they've been all wrong about *who* smokes weed (which is true, of course), I think we need to focus on the far more significant fact that they've been all wrong about weed itself. Way wrong! Unbelievably, terribly, *catastrophically* wrong!

And the first people they owe an apology to for this are the very "stoners" Ms. Mannix wants to oh-so-cleverly *weed out.* The type of losers who wear pot-leaf T-shirts, forward emails about how hemp can help reverse climate change, and keep going on and on about how cannabis might save your life if you've got cancer, epilepsy, or countless other conditions. You know, the total burnouts who spent decades tirelessly pushing marijuana legalization as a political issue without the support of corporate America, the unions, special interests, or either major party. And most especially the ones who risked arrest and imprisonment as growers and distributors to make sure the rest of us could get high.

But if you're waiting for an apology from the powers that be for the War on Pot, don't hold your breath. Despite all the dramatic change of the last decade, such mea culpas have been few and far between. CNN's Dr. Sanjay Gupta came closest to hitting the mark in 2013, telling millions of viewers around the world, "We have been terribly and systematically misled for nearly seventy years in the United States, and I apologize for my own role in that."

Specifically, Gupta admitted to ignoring studies conducted outside the United States that showed cannabis's tremendous healing properties; trusting the government's pronouncements on the drug's purported dangers without examining the underlying science; and being "too dismissive of the loud chorus of legitimate patients whose symptoms improved on cannabis."

Now think about that last line for a minute, and you'll understand just how deep the prejudice against this plant runs. Dr. Gupta didn't miss a hidden clue on a few obscure cases that could have pointed to marijuana's healing properties, if only he'd made the connection. No, by his own account, he dismissed a "loud chorus" of "legitimate patients," some of whom literally walked right up to him and said, "My symptoms improve when I use cannabis." Then he ignored peer-reviewed scientific studies that proved them right—at a time when, as a leading figure in both the media and the medical establishment, he could have helped save countless lives and relieved untold pain and suffering by sharing that information. All because he apparently thought so little of marijuana users that he believed large numbers of us would make up stories about miraculously healing ourselves.

Despite all that, I haven't met a single medical-cannabis patient or activist who doesn't readily, happily, graciously accept Dr. Gupta's apology. After all, we pretty much invented taking the high road when it comes to these sorts of things.

Seize the Jay

I'm pleased to report that the tired old Cheech and Chong trope of a lazy, burned-out stoner sitting in his parents' basement with a bong and zero ambition no longer appears in every single portrayal of cannabis culture on TV and in the movies. And I say that with no disrespect to Cheech Marin and Tommy Chong themselves, or the films and albums they've made together, all of which actually satirize the idea that marijuana turns you into a pathetic loser in a way that's both really funny and deeply subversive.

Still, if you find yourself occasionally hitting the bong and then succumbing to what psychologists call "amotivational syndrome" (and stoners call "couch lock"), kindly consider following my foolproof, three-step plan for getting off your ass, and utilizing your high—every time, guaranteed. *Carpe Diesel!*

> **STEP 1:** Decide what you're going to do *after* you get stoned, *before* you get stoned.
>
> **STEP 2:** Get stoned.
>
> **STEP 3:** Do whatever you decided on in step 1.

CANNABIS CUSTOMS

Ceremonies, customs, and rituals all play a vital role in keeping the cannabis community connected, vital, and continuous. Learn them well, and pass them on . . .

- When sharing in a group, pass a joint, blunt, bowl, bong, or other smoking device to the left, as a reminder to literally and figuratively follow your heart.

- Don't Bogart that joint, my friend! (Meaning don't hog the herb without passing, the way film legend Humphrey Bogart let a cigarette perpetually dangle from his lower lip.)

- Never disparage someone else's pot, or refuse to smoke it in favor of your own.

- When supplies run low in a shared stash situation, make sure you're extra-efficient with the herb.

- Don't *bongtificate* (that is, treat a joint, bowl, or bong like it's a microphone and just talk and talk while everybody else waits their turn to smoke).

- There's a time and place for gravity bongs, and it's called college.

- If you're smoking someone else's weed, be respectful of the fact that they're gifting you something wonderful (not to mention pricey). If someone else is smoking your stash, don't act like that suddenly makes you lord of the manor.

⚕ Never, ever, ever pretend to be the fucking cops!

⚕ Don't judge people who smoke more than you or less than you.

⚕ Never "out" a closeted cannabis user, even accidentally. And this includes in states where it's perfectly legal.

⚕ Avoid compromising the integrity of someone else's high. Which means that if your smoking buddy wants to turn cartwheels, play the bongos, or make a peanut-butter-and-banana hemp-milk smoothie, either join in or find something else to do.

HOW TO THROW A
WEED-THEMED DINNER PARTY

Why waste another night going out and spending too much money on booze and coat checks when you can cook an amazing meal at home, get blazed with all your friends, and then settle in for an evening of marijuana-infused merriment?

Start by carefully planning your guest list, remembering what the Dude said: *There's an art to hanging, and it starts with who you're hanging with.*

So make a tally of all your friends who really like to toke and then decide how many of them you'd realistically want to entertain in your home at once. For a dinner party, it's best to keep it to eight or fewer to ensure an intimate vibe. Also, rather than arranging an evening where everyone knows one another already, mix and match from the compartments of your life. And don't try to guess how different people (Susie from kickboxing class, Fred from high school) will get along in advance or worry over who has "nothing in common," because you'd be surprised how quickly and irrevocably the herb can break the ice between otherwise disparate temperaments once things "get rolling."

At the appointed hour, greet each new arrival with a relaxed smile, plenty of comfortable seating, upbeat, instrumental music at a moderate volume, and two well-appointed tables—one covered in ready-to-eat light snacks, the other home to a collection of labeled jars of cannabis and concentrates, plus a few empty jars and blank labels so guests can add a bit of their own herb to the communal stash. Take time to point out all the strains thus assembled and what you know about them while encouraging everyone else to do the same for their own offerings. Then let all heads decide for themselves how and when to dig in using the wide array of rolling papers, filters, grinders, pipes, and vaporizers you've thoughtfully provided alongside the jars.

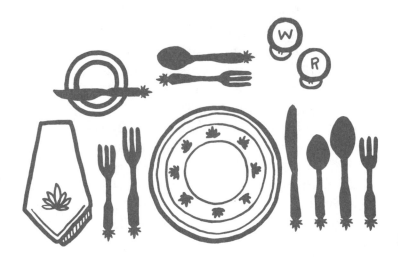

As for the dinner part of this dinner party, how you approach preparing the main course should depend on your general level of culinary competence and your guests' expectations. In any case, stick with a menu of dishes you've made successfully before, since you'll be scaling them up significantly to feed all your super-stoned friends while operating in a thick haze of marijuana smoke.

Basically, "cook with your head, not over it," as I put it in a VICE Weed Eater column titled "The Joy of Cooking (While Really Stoned)"—in which I also suggested that "to fully experience the joy of cooking while *really* stoned, first attain basic proficiency in both of those disciplines separately before ever attempting to combine them." Additional relevant advice included "limit multitasking," "always set timers," and "use the buddy system whenever possible." This last bit of guidance is especially helpful for a large dinner party, as you'll most definitely want a co-conspirator to help you with cooking, setting up, serving, and (sigh) cleaning up the mess left behind.

For that particular column, I enlisted the expert assistance of chef Gabriel Reeves, a ten-year veteran of fine-dining kitchens who now works at Elemental Wellness Center—one of California's top medical-cannabis dispensaries—where he teaches a popular weekly pot-cooking class, prepares daily healthy non-medicated lunches for a staff of forty, and advises patients on using medical marijuana effectively.

"I've learned three things about stoned diners," Chef Gabe revealed at the outset of our menu-planning session, "ranch dressing, Tabasco sauce, and gravy. When you've got the munchies, ketchup, mustard, and mayo are all *eh*. But if I serve you an empty clamshell full of broken glass covered in a nicely made gravy, with Tabasco and ranch on the side, that's game over. And every cuisine has some version of that, whether it's the classic French sauces, fish sauce, or curry."

Wise words to keep in mind as you plan *your* menu. Also look for dishes that can be prepared in advance, so you'll have more time to get stoned and hang heavy with your guests, rather than taking care of last-minute kitchen tasks. Perhaps you can even organize a round or two of Jenga or Pictionary to keep spirits high during the snacking hour. Just don't wait too long to serve the main course, or your more lightweight guests may subtly start slipping from pleasantly faded to irrevocably couch locked.

THE HIGH HOLIDAYS

Every year on April 20 (4/20), marijuana lovers celebrate their favorite plant with festivals, concerts, marches, and smoke-outs great and small. So what are the origins of this high holiday, and how best to mark the occasion?

Way back in 2008, I appeared on NPR to answer those questions and many others. But first, along with the show's hosts, I helped dispel some common misconceptions about the 420 phenomenon. For instance, April 20 is not Jerry Garcia's birthday, nor is it the day Jimi Hendrix died. British high tea is not served precisely at 4:20 P.M., and there are not 420 psychoactive chemicals in cannabis—nor is 420 the official police code for marijuana smoking in progress.

"The true story," I explained to a national radio audience, "is actually stranger and nicer than any of the legends . . ."

The original 420 code started among a small group of friends in the 1970s in San Rafael, California, who would get together to smoke pot every day at 4:20 in the afternoon under a statue of Louis Pasteur. San Rafael was the headquarters of the Grateful Dead's business operations at the time, so the tradition sort of got passed along informally through the Deadhead network when the band went out on tour. And from there, 420 went global, because it served a vital purpose. Every oppressed, underground subculture needs a discreet way to self-identify.

Of course, once the squares started to crack our code, it no longer served that original function effectively, so we made up a new one. Now on 4/20, every year, marijuana enthusiasts enjoy a huge day of celebration. And it's a great thing for this culture to have a holiday set aside where we can be proud of ourselves and show the world what we are all about.

For me, that rapid transformation of 420—from an underground bit of in-the-know slang to an all-out loud-and-proud public celebration of cannabis culture—represents the recent tidal shift in public opinion in America regarding marijuana better than anything else. Now, as far as how best to celebrate all that social and political progress, the important factor isn't where you choose to mark the occasion—from the world's biggest smoke-out to a quiet inner-circle session out in the woods—it's making sure that you take the opportunity, at least that once a year, to stop and smell the Kush, so to speak.

Sure, you're likely going to smoke a little (or a lot) more weed than usual on 4/20, and that's probably as it should be, but don't fall into the St. Patrick's Day trap of making overconsumption into some kind of cherished annual tradition. Instead, slow your roll just a bit, and make time to reflect with some depth on the important role this plant plays in your life and the lives of many millions of people around the world. Then make a list of those you enjoy sharing cannabis with the most and invite them over, set up a Skype session, or plan some kind of special group outing.

Just don't forget that while your own cannabis cup runneth over, many others still live in want, need, or outright herbal oppression. I was reminded of this the year 4/20 fell on the first night of Passover, just a couple of days after I'd appeared on NPR—a coincidence of the calendar that naturally gave way to a string of jokes about whether or not pot's kosher (it is!) and when, exactly, to partake of "the less bitter herb."

When I observed Passover with my family that year, however, and together we recounted the story of how an oppressed people gained their freedom, I couldn't help but notice certain more serious parallels to the plight of the pot tribe. So perhaps the ceremonies surrounding our high holiday should reflect the same mix of deliverance, defiance, and determination that Jews adopt when looking back at their own moment of liberation. In particular, I was struck by the parts of the ritualistic Passover meal known as a seder where all assembled pour out a bit of their wine (*way* before NWA did it) in recognition of those who lived their whole lives as slaves, those who died on the journey out of bondage, and even those among the oppressors who drowned in the Red Sea.

And so, each year, on 4/20, I take a moment amid the marijuana madness to grind up one small (OK, *very* small) perfect little bud and then set it adrift on the wind. At which point I usually let some very enthusiastic person talk me into hitting one of those giant five-ounce megajoints that people roll up at 4:20 on 4/20, even though I'd really rather not. After all, 4/20 only comes around once a year!

Oil's Well

Write the number 710 out as if it were on the face of an old-school digital alarm clock, then flip it upside down. Spoiler alert: it spells "OIL." And that, plus the Internet, brings us 7/10 or (July 10), a relatively new high holiday dedicated specifically to smoking butane honey oil and other types of dabs.

🌿 PRO TIP 🌿

TIMING IS EVERYTHING

"I used to smoke marijuana. But I'll tell you something: I would only smoke it in the late evening. Oh, occasionally the early evening, but usually the late evening—or the midevening. Just the early evening, midevening, and late evening. Occasionally, early afternoon, early midafternoon, or perhaps the late-midafternoon. Oh, sometimes the early-mid-late-early morning. . . . But never at dusk."

—STEVE MARTIN, *A WILD AND CRAZY GUY*

"I smoke a lot of pot, but only when all work is done and just a puff or two as a treat. . . . I have [also] found if I smoke a little pot before I play basketball I become amazing and hear myself saying things like 'not on my watch' a lot."

—SARAH SILVERMAN, IN AN INTERVIEW WITH ANDY BOROWITZ

BEGINNER'S MIND:
HOW DYLAN TURNED ON THE BEATLES

Even the great and exalted Bob Marley once smoked ganja for the first time. And he probably asked a bunch of dumb questions and coughed too much throughout. So if you're ever called upon to help guide an uninitiated friend or relative into the wonderful world of herbal delights, you must strive to remain exceedingly patient, kind, and accommodating throughout the proceedings—no matter what. Remember, "Doob unto Others." Also, make sure your friend's potentially auspicious first puff takes place in a comfortable, safe, familiar setting, ideally among a small group of close friends. And don't ever let things get overly uptight or (conversely) totally freaked-out—not for the initiate, or for you.

After all, getting someone high for the first time is both a great privilege and a serious responsibility, not to mention an excellent opportunity to recall the heady feeling of your own early days in the herb game. So rather than coming on as some kind of guru or guide, just relax, let nature run its course, and try to recapture a bit of your own "beginner's mind" when it comes to marijuana. If you can achieve that exalted plane, you just might end up having a transcendent journey of your own.

"It's my experience that to smoke marijuana for the first time is to explore the limits of hilarity only to find that there are no limits," famed music journalist Al Aronowitz once noted, an observation eerily reminiscent of my own first time behind the bowling alley. "You laugh so hard that you want to laugh that hard again, so you smoke marijuana again. And again and again and again and again. I'm told that few ever really succeed in laughing that hard a second time, but I did. The two biggest laughs of my life were the first time I smoked marijuana and the first time the Beatles smoked it."

Aronowitz didn't "turn on" the Beatles (who later used "let's go have a laugh" as their private code for getting high) so much as he introduced them to Bob Dylan, who gladly did the honors. The deal went down on August 28, 1964, at New York City's swanky Delmonico Hotel. Upon arrival, Dylan mistakenly believed the Beatles—whom he was meeting for the first time—already smoked grass, based on a misheard lyric on "I Want to Hold Your Hand." Leaving John Lennon to bashfully point out that the lads from Liverpool were actually singing "I can't hide," not "I get high," on the chorus.

From there, a scene unfolded straight out of a B-movie stoner comedy, only it starred some of the twentieth century's most influential and enduring artists at the very outset of their storied careers. According to Aronowitz's lengthy first-person account of the encounter in his book *Bob Dylan and the Beatles*:

> *The Beatles wanted to know how the marijuana would make them feel and we told them it would make them feel good. I still hadn't learned how to roll a joint in those days, so when the Beatles agreed to try some, I asked Dylan to roll the first joint. Bob wasn't much of a roller either, and a lot of the grass fell into the big bowl of fruit on the room service table.*

Dylan first offered the joint to John Lennon, but the group's unofficial leader immediately handed it to Ringo, demanding the drummer serve as the other Beatles' "royal taster"—ostensibly to make sure the drug didn't prove poisonous or provoke insanity before the rest committed to trying it. So Ringo started inhaling. At which point the first Beatle to get high immediately (though unwittingly) committed one of the very few major pot faux pas we outlined earlier, as Aronowitz explains:

As Ringo kept taking hits, Bob and I waited for him to pass the joint to John, who was sitting right next to Ringo. But the Beatles were unacquainted with the rituals of pot smoking. Pot smokers share joints because it's precious stuff. It's illegal, expensive and not easy to get. Pot smokers don't waste any smoke letting the joint burn idly like a cigarette. . . . I neglected to instruct Ringo about passing the joint and it was obvious that he was going to hold onto it as if he were smoking a cigarette filled with tobacco. I didn't want to risk the possibility that the Beatles might recoil from the idea of passing a joint from lips to lips like a bottle shared by winos on a street corner.

A delicate moment indeed, which Aronowitz ably resolved by asking Dylan's rolling-adept road manager to quickly produce a few more joints, until everybody had one of their own. Then, since Ringo had gotten a head start on getting high, he started to feel the effects first, and unleashed a ripple of laughter that quickly reverberated throughout the room.

Soon, Ringo got the giggles. In no time at all, he was laughing hysterically. His laughing looked so funny that the rest of us started laughing hysterically. . . . We kept laughing at one another's laughter until every one of us had been laughed at. There also came a certain point when Paul realized he was really thinking for the first time in his life and he also realized that this was a great occasion. He told [Beatles road manager] Mal Evans to get a pad and a pen and to write down everything he said.

Unfortunately, more than fifty years later, that historic document either remains in private hands or has been lost to history forever. But what we do know is that shortly after their fateful encounter with Bob Dylan, the Beatles would start to rapidly transform their music from the teenybopper bubblegum pop

sound that made them global sensations into the more experimental, expansive, psychedelic explorations that kick-started
the social and political upheaval of the '60s and helped usher
marijuana into the mainstream. All because Al Aronowitz made
every effort imaginable to ensure that the Fab Four's first time
getting high went smoothly, despite a lot of awkward tension in
the room as the world's biggest music stars took great pains to
show each other proper deference.

"Allen Ginsberg would afterwards ask me if this initial
meeting between Bob and the Beatles was *demure*," Aronowitz
wrote, "and that is exactly the right word for it." At least until
things broke out into a spontaneous, all-encompassing five-way
laughing fit.

Ginsberg, the famed beat poet, author of *Howl*, and running
buddy of Jack Kerouac, by the way, also put great stock in personal insights gained the first time he got high—as he much later
explained to Larry "Ratso" Sloman in his 1998 book *Reefer
Madness.*

*When I smoked grass [the first time] I suddenly realized how
amazing it was that on the evidence of my own senses, which I
did not doubt, here was a very mild stimulator of perception
that led me into all sorts of awes and cosmic vibrations and ap-
preciations of Cézanne and Renaissance paintings and color and
tastes. And here was this great big government plot to suppress
it and make it seem as if it were something diabolic, satanic, full
of hatred and fiendishness and madness. . . . It was the very first
time I ever had solid evidence in my own body that there was a
difference between reality as I saw it myself and reality as it was
described officially by the state, the government, the police and
the media. From then on I realized that marijuana was going to
be an enormous political catalyst, because anybody who got high
would immediately see through the official hallucination that*

had been laid down and would begin questioning, "What is this War? What is the military budget?"

That powerful realization led Ginsberg to cofound America's first pro-marijuana lobbying and activism organization and become a lifelong advocate for not just cannabis liberation but for the demise of repressive regimes around the world. He also conspired with author Norman Mailer to hijack a live episode of a national television talk show and use it as a platform for America's first substantial fact-based discussion of marijuana in a public forum since the herb was made federally illegal in the 1930s.

Mailer, though less enthusiastic than Ginsberg, agreed to the plan in honor of his own reverence for the herb. In a *Paris Review* interview, the controversial, iconoclastic novelist once claimed that his lifelong habit of intense self-analysis "started with marijuana because I found that, smoking marijuana, I became real to myself for the first time." He later described to *High Times* a more sensual herbal epiphany that struck him the very first time he got high:

> *I was out in the car listening to the radio. Some jazz came on. I'd been listening to jazz for years, but it had never meant all that much to me. Now, with the powers pot offered, simple things became complex; complex things clarified themselves. These musicians were offering the inner content of their experiences to me.*

So, to recap: When the Beatles tried pot for the first time, they metamorphosed from a hard-drinking, pill-popping commercially oriented boy band into harbingers of a coming peacenik psychedelic revolution; when Allen Ginsberg got high, he started questioning authority and exploring the illegitimacy of the government; and Norman Mailer's first dance with Mary Jane offered powerful insights into himself that, somewhat paradoxically, also opened him up to an empathic understanding of another culture's art and experience.

No wonder the powers that be are afraid of this herb!

TRAIL GUIDE: HOW TO GET A FRIEND HIGH (PROPERLY) FOR THE FIRST TIME

Combine a steady hand on the wheel with a healthy sense of adventure when riding copilot on someone else's maiden marijuana voyage.

- ⚕ Never pressure someone to try cannabis for the first time (or the tenth time) unless you believe they need it for serious health reasons.

- ⚕ Don't let someone try marijuana for the first time if they're already intoxicated on alcohol (or other drugs), as this combination may prove highly unpleasant in the short term ("Have you ever puked your guts out, *on weed*?") and could also result in your pot protégé swearing off ever trying the herb again.

- ⚕ Turn all cell phones off for the duration. Instead, take a tip from Paul McCartney and have a good old-fashioned notebook on hand, to write down your best *high*-deas for later contemplation.

- ⚕ Prior to lift-off, encourage any new initiate to first learn as much as possible about cannabis, which will both

help them better appreciate the experience and also ease
any fears they may have about what's about to happen.

⚜ For experienced users, cannabis serves best as an enhancement of life's many pleasures, like going to a ga-
rage sale or playing a vigorous game of volleyball, but
remember that newbies may feel a little overwhelmed,
antisocial, or even unsteady on their feet when the
herb hits them for the first time. So choose a private
location with plenty of comfortable seating, mellow
lighting, nice music, and an *irie* vibration, where you
won't be disturbed by anyone or anything that could
potentially compromise the integrity of your high.

⚜ Since THC works primarily by interacting with the
body's natural endocannabinoid system, it sometimes
takes naïve users several attempts to ingest enough to
start feeling the effects. That said, it's still important to
go slow. Remember, you can always get higher, but
you can't always get less high (at least not in a hurry).

⚜ Hydrate immediately before and after those first few
puffs. Cottonmouth kills—your buzz!

⚜ If possible, have some CBD-rich cannabis on hand,
ideally as a tincture, as that will help quickly "bring
down" someone experiencing an unpleasant THC
high. Smoking CBD-rich buds will have the same effect, but it may be tough to convince someone enduring a freak-out that smoking *more* pot is the answer.

⚜ When the magic moment at last arrives, you go first.
Take two quick, shallow puffs into your lungs and

then exhale immediately. (Holding in smoke in any longer doesn't get you higher, but will lead to coughing fits, especially for newbies, and potential irritation of the lungs.)

* Once you've shown the way, have your initiate follow suit by taking in the smallest amount of smoke possible, and working up from there. Then, after a couple of solid exhales, put the herb down and wait at least ten minutes to gauge the effects (if any). Repeat as necessary until you both get high, or run out of weed.

* Whatever happens next, don't judge, don't shame, and impose no restrictions unless you fear harm to yourselves or others (for example, no driving). Otherwise, go with the flow and let the chips fall where they may.

PRO TIP

YOU'RE NOT THE FIRST PERSON TO GET HIGH FOR THE FIRST TIME

MAYA ANGELOU,
FROM *GATHER TOGETHER IN MY NAME*
San Diego, California, Mid-1940s

I had smoked cigarettes for over a year, but never marijuana. But since I had the unmitigated gall to sit up cross-legged in a lesbian apartment sipping wine, I felt I had the stamina to smoke a little grita.

I opened my throat and kept my tongue flat so that the smoke found no obstacle in its passage from my lips to my throat. It tore the lining off my tonsils, made my nasal passages burn like red pepper, and choked me. While I coughed, gagging, those silly bitches laughed. . . . Wouldn't they do anything for me? No. Beatrice rescued the joint and sucked in the smoke, puffing out her already fat cheeks to bursting, while her lady love was busily engaged in rolling another stick of tearing fire.

The food was the best I ever tasted. Every morsel was an experience of sheer delight. I lost myself in a haze of sensual pleasure, enjoying not only the tastes, but the feel of the food in my mouth, the smells, and the sound of my jaws chewing.

WILLIE NELSON,
FROM *WILLIE: AN AUTOBIOGRAPHY*
Ft. Worth, Texas, 1954

Marijuana was known as tea or reefer or weed or boo. . . . Fred [Lockwood] and I had been sitting in some saloon watching the Army-McCarthy hearings on black-and-white TV and listening to Doris Day singing "Hey There" on the jukebox when he suggested we blow tea. After I turned him down, he gave me a skinny little joint with both ends twisted and told me to get high and be somebody.

On the way home, I pulled my car to the side of the road and lit up. I smoked the whole joint and waited for something to happen. I had puffed the joint and blown out the smoke, not taking the smoke all the way down and holding it like you're supposed to. I didn't even get a little bit high. I thought: What's the big deal? If I want to get high and be somebody, I'll drink a quart of bourbon. For six months I bummed joints now and then from Fred and puffed them and still didn't get high.

Finally one night I did it right. Since then, I have made up for those wasted six months.

DAVID BOWIE,
FROM AN INTERVIEW IN *PLAYBOY*
London, Mid-1960s

The first time I got stoned on grass was with John Paul Jones of Led Zeppelin, when he was still a bass player on Herman's Hermits records. . . . Jonesy said to me, "Come over and I'll turn you on to grass." I thought about it and said, "Sure, I'll give it a whirl." We went over to his flat—he had a huge room, with nothing in it except this huge vast Hammond organ—right next door to the police department.

I watched in wonder while Jonesy rolled these three fat joints. And we got stoned on all of them. I became incredibly high and it turned into an in-fucking-credible hunger. I ate two loaves of bread. Then the telephone rang. Jonesy said, "Go and answer that for me, will you?" So I went downstairs to answer the phone and kept on walking right out into the street. I never went back.

WHAT TO DO (AND NOT DO)
IF YOU'RE TOO DAMN HIGH IN PUBLIC

Knowing what to do if you're too high in private is easy. Just stay calm, stay hydrated, and find a quiet, dimly lit place to lie down and wait out the storm. But what if you go one toke over the line while "sitting downtown in the railway station," as in the classic song by Brewer and Shipley?

Well, that's a different story. Staying calm and staying hydrated still apply, but there's certainly no quiet, dimly lit place you'll want to lie down at the railway station. So it's time to work on something seasoned pot smokers call *maintaining*. But first, take note that an ounce of prevention truly is worth a pound of cure in these cases, meaning the easiest way to deal with getting too high in public is to not get high in public in the first place. Especially if you're a fairly inexperienced herbalist, or you find that ingesting THC sometimes triggers feelings of anxiety. After all, smoking pot is supposed to be fun, not a harrowing ordeal.

That said, it happens to the best of us. One minute you're ripping a vape pen full of concentrates outside the station, to kill a little time while waiting for your train, the next you're staring at the departure board with a bone-dry mouth and a brain full of panic. Some part of this reaction is clearly physiological, as large doses of THC can produce disorientation and dissociative feelings, while some is also clearly psychological, and largely attributable to marijuana's illicit nature. Because, really, people would say avocados made them paranoid if 600,000 Americans got arrested for eating guacamole every year. And the guy you buy your tacos from just might be a snitch.

Anyway, in the hypothetical railway-station scenario, it would be relatively easy to maintain. Simply stay in one place, take deep breaths, watch carefully for the announcement of your train, board your train, and sit down—in a window seat if possible—all while picturing your happy place. Get your train ticket ready long before the conductor arrives, and keep all conversation to the barest pleasantries. All in all, just play it cool and pretty soon you should start feeling better.

But what if your bout of green panic sets in at a social function—say, at a family wedding? One minute you and a few of the cool cousins are hotboxing a Chevy Impala out in the parking lot, the next you're getting jiggy on the dance floor when the DJ turns on a giant strobe light, and everything disintegrates like fractals in a blender.

Again, stay calm, and stay hydrated, but you can't exactly stay in one place and wait things out this time. So step one is getting away from the dance music and flashing lights—quickly, but without hurrying. Rushing out of the room will only make things worse inside your head, plus you might run into something (or someone), and people will stare. An all-around poor outcome.

Also, don't ever flee to the bathroom, unless you feel an urgent physical need to relieve yourself. Otherwise, that's the last place you're going to feel comforted and at peace. Instead, head for the nearest fresh air you can find. Odds are, a few minutes of alone time in the great outdoors and you'll turn the corner. And when you come back, if anyone asks, just say you had to take a private phone call—if that sounds plausible—or that you had too much to drink and needed to fend off the spins if everyone noticed you looked a little fucked-up on the way out.

HOW TO DEAL WITH ALCOHOL CULTURE

My good friend and VICE colleague T. Kid writes a weekly column called Weediquette that explores both the personal and the political when it comes to smoking pot, all in his inimitably introspective style. One week he spins a wild yarn about getting his aunt high for the first time in a few decades, and the next he's asking, "Did Obama just screw weed legalization by supporting it?"

So when he posted a Weediquette under the headline "I Like to Stay Home," I honestly expected something sort of silly, perhaps an ode to the joys of the couch, pizza delivery, and Netflix. Instead, he got to the heart of an issue so big most of us can't really see it. Namely, the fact that we live in an absolutely alcohol-soaked culture. He wrote:

> The central point of socialization in most places of the world is alcohol. Sporting, coupling, celebration, sympathy, relaxation, and just about every other social institution, save for AA, is accompanied by drinking. In college I was as limitless in my capacity for alcohol as any 21-year-old, but ... just after I graduated from college, I was out drinking, positively shitfaced, with a friend in Baltimore when we were jumped by a gang of boys trying to steal our cell phones. One of them stabbed me in the throat with a broken glass bottle.

For the next year, T. Kid stayed sequestered at his parents' house, smoking tons of weed to kill the pain of a severed nerve. In time, he physically recovered, but "alcohol never, ever felt the same." And when it came time to leave the nest again, he discovered that quitting drinking in favor of weed meant stepping almost wholly outside the mainstream of society, to the point that it often felt better to just stay home.

I resumed my social life but began to see every engagement as a chore. The comfort that I had felt as an agoraphobe [while recovering] never left my temperament, and I would watch the clock any time I was out, waiting for the right moment to make an exit. . . . As my drinking diminished to nothing, my friends grew into real Philadelphia men, for whom drinking was a consistent habit. Overworked, embittered, and slowly being crushed by the responsibilities of the real world, their beer bellies grew, and to this day those paunches remain monuments to their owners' desperation for escape.

Without belaboring an obvious point, it's total insanity that (addictive, destructive, deadly) alcohol is literally the basis for almost every social interaction in our society—including a "beer summit" organized by the president of the United States as a way to help ease tensions between African Americans and the police—while, for more than a century, a whole global community of peace-loving people has been forcibly prevented from congregating together to share their own sacrament.

Which sort of makes you rethink the tired old stereotype of lazy stoners sitting on the couch wasting their lives away, doesn't it? Maybe we just don't like hanging out with a bunch of loudmouthed drunks—or getting arrested, for that matter.

And remember, it hasn't always been this way. Back in the 1930s, before marijuana was made federally illegal, the herb's early adopters used to gather together at after-hours places called "tea pads" that cropped up after the jazz clubs closed. In addition to a swinging place to get high and hear the scene's best musicians at their most intimate and uninhibited, tea pads also served as a neutral space where men and women, black and white, young and old, of all economic means and political persuasions, could meet, unwind, intermingle, and exchange ideas away from polite society's disapproving eyes.

In 1938, the *New Yorker*'s Meyer Berger dedicated weeks of legwork to tracking down one of these underground cannabis clubs. In "Tea for a Viper," he gained entrée to Chappy's, a dark, austere spot in Harlem with music, muggles (jazz slang for weed), and dancing till dawn. After getting to know the regulars, Berger became convinced that the reefer madness tales of the day didn't hold up to close observation.

Federal agents told me that vipers are always dangerous; that an overdose of marijuana generates savage and sadistic traits likely to reach a climax in axe and icepick murders. . . . Medical experts seem to agree that marijuana, while no more habit-forming than ordinary cigarette smoking, offers a shorter cut to complete madness than any other drug. They say it causes deterioration of the brain. Chappy's customers scoffed at this idea. They said reefers only made them happy. They didn't know a single viper who was vicious or mad.

In 1944, a blue-ribbon report on marijuana commissioned by New York City mayor Fiorello La Guardia further described the phenomenon:

A "tea-pad" is a room or an apartment in which people gather to smoke marihuana. . . . The lighting is more or less uniformly dim, with blue predominating. An incense is considered part of the furnishings. . . .

The marihuana smoker derives greater satisfaction [when] smoking in the presence of others. His attitude in the "tea-pad" is that of a relaxed individual, free from the anxieties and cares of the realities of life. The "tea-pad" takes on the atmosphere of a very congenial social club. The smoker readily engages in conversation with strangers, discussing freely his pleasant reactions to the drug and philosophizing on subjects pertaining to life in a manner which, at times, appears to be out of keeping with his intellectual level. A constant observation was the extreme willingness to share and puff on each other's cigarettes.

Which means seemingly agoraphobic stoners don't actually *want* to stay home all the time, they're just waiting for someone to open a 420-friendly spot that *"takes on the atmosphere of a very congenial social club."*

For decades, Amsterdam's coffeeshops have been doing just that, with the best ones exuding the Dutch sense of *gezellig*—an untranslatable word at the heart of the national identity that roughly means "coziness." I'll never forget my first trip to the Netherlands, including the sensation of liberation I experienced walking into a coffeeshop and ordering my herb off a legit menu. Rather quickly one grows accustomed to being treated like a customer instead of a criminal, but that first time was actually very emotional. I got a hot chocolate with whipped cream along with a gram each of Neville's Haze bud and some Moroccan hash, then sat down at a booth near the window to take it all in.

I've returned to that same coffeeshop many times since, and that's still my regular order: haze, hash, and hot chocolate. Not just because it's a pretty fucking epic combination, but also to remind myself of that first trip, and the profound feeling that came over me while looking around at the other patrons, and sharing knowing smiles even with those with whom I shared no other common language. We'd each made a pilgrimage to Amsterdam from around the world not to smoke weed—we'd all done that hundreds of times at home—but to sit down and light up with the same rights as someone who'd rather duck into a bar across the street for a cold beer.

Like the La Guardia report said, *"The marihuana smoker derives greater satisfaction [when] smoking in the presence of others."*

WHEN SHARING BECOMES MOOCHING

Money's always a touchy subject, and often more so when it comes to marijuana, since it's something most people want to share freely, even though it's hardly free. So here are some basic guidelines for when it comes time to divvy up the stash.

- ⚕ Never ask a casual acquaintance or an occasional (once a week or less) pot smoker to throw in on your herb unless you're in dire straits. If they want to be polite, or balance the scales, just let them buy you a slice of pizza or some other small *tokin'* of appreciation after the session. But a direct cash remuneration for a one-time, small-scale sharing of marijuana is tacky, awkward, and outside good taste.

- ⚕ If someone consistently imposes on your generosity by sharing your cannabis, without ever returning the favor (directly or indirectly), feel free to be honest about your feelings, but wait to do so until you can speak to the person privately, when neither of you are blazed. And rather than taking a confrontational approach, try simply mentioning that your weed budget has been getting stretched a little thin lately, and perhaps there's a way to make things a bit more equitable.

- ⚕ Always be clear on the difference between a communal stash (which everybody throws in on) and a personal stash (which one person buys and then decides to share), and then get all related financial transactions squared away *before* you start smoking.

☀ A ganja session is like the dinner table—not an appropriate place to discuss money. Feel free to get into religion and politics, though.

☀ Sad to say, but unless you're ill, if you're smoking more marijuana than you can afford, you must either cut back or get a better-paying job. Because unlike Blanche DuBois in *A Streetcar Named Desire,* you can't always rely on the kindness of strangers. Or even your best buds.

RISE UP, FREEDOM FIGHTERS

Smoking pot properly requires more than just knowing how to twist up a joint in a windstorm. Duty also requires working meaningfully toward cannabis freedom for one and all. And that's especially true for those of us lucky enough to live in a place where marijuana's already legal or available legally to those with a doctor's recommendation. After all, it's understandable for herbalists stuck in places where the plant's heavily repressed to shy away from speaking up publicly. So the onus is on the rest of us to get up, stand up, and demand equal rights for all!

☀ Start by learning everything possible about this wonderful plant in all its aspects. Read about marijuana (you're doing that right now!), watch documentaries, absorb marijuana culture, and talk to educated friends about marijuana until you understand the herb's social, political, botanical, medicinal, industrial, and spiritual uses; the history of its cultivation and consumption; the dark forces behind prohibition; and the many benefits of legalization.

⚝ Make contact with the grassroots cannabis activism community by attending a meeting of your local chapter of NORML—the National Organization for the Reform of Marijuana Laws—or another reform group that suits your fancy (see page 141). Not only is "acting locally" the key to ending the global War on Weed, getting directly involved in the marijuana movement also feels great and will introduce you to some fascinating new friends who share a common interest.

⚝ When appropriate, use social media to spread targeted pro-cannabis messages designed to positively influence others in your network, rather than simply get the most likes. Which means a thoughtful meme contrasting the health risks of consuming the food at McDonald's (terrible!) to those of smoking pot (health-positive!) works wonders, while posting about the time you got high and couldn't find your sunglasses for an hour, not so much. Also, never, ever share anything incriminating (to yourself or others) on social media in any form.

⚝ Contact your elected officials—local, state, and federal—and make sure they know that you're a taxpayer and a voter who believes strongly in marijuana legalization as an issue of personal liberty, fiscal responsibility, and common sense. Sign up for "action alerts" from norml.org and other reform groups so you can follow up with specific lawmakers when marijuana issues come before the government.

⚝ Attend cannabis seminars and events that aim to educate both enthusiasts and the general public about the plant in a fun, responsible manner. Aside from all the good vibes of joining a cannabis-centric crowd, there's also a truly heady feeling that comes with knowing you're far from alone in believing that this is an important issue.

* Make a pilgrimage to a state with full marijuana legalization for all adults, and document your trip in detail, including visits to marijuana stores, a cultivation facility, and other aspects of the local cannabis culture. Then share your journey with as many friends, family, and acquaintances as possible, so they can see the benefits of making marijuana a taxed and regulated part of the aboveground economy, rather than pushing it into the black market.

* Study the most common arguments used against legalization, and figure out how to respond in advance. Because once you start speaking up for Mary Jane, you're going to hear the same old bullshit over and over, from the "gateway theory," to "pot is way stronger than it used to be," to "stoned driving," "What about the children?" and "THC gummy bears." So like a chess player, you've got to have all the basic moves and countermoves gamed out in advance, before the real battle even begins.

* Support only cannabis organizations and businesses that exhibit the plant's true values, including honesty, transparency, compassion, equality, inclusion, kindness, and peace. Help build a progressive marijuana industry by helping those who do it right flourish and grow.

✿ If you have the means, consider writing a check to your favorite marijuana-law-reform organization. Right now, the public strongly backs legalization, but the movement still needs sufficient funding to push the issue and take full advantage of this historic shift in public sentiment.

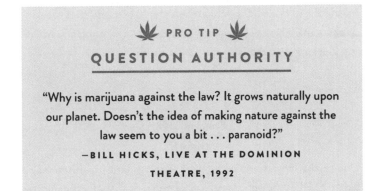

MARIJUANA ORGS

There's never been a better time to get up, stand up for every adult's right to grow, possess, and consume cannabis—in all forms, and for any reason—than right now. And there's also never been more high-quality marijuana-law-reform organizations working on this vital social-justice issue, each with a unique approach. So do some research, find the one that's right for you, and then get in touch and ask them how you can become a stakeholder in your own liberation.

NORML
Founded: 1971

norml.org

The nation's oldest and largest organization advocating marijuana legalization, NORML has thousands of active members and hundreds of local chapters spread all across the United States and around the world. Find the chapter closest to you, and start speaking up about marijuana policy where you live, while meeting new friends and plugging in to the local cannabis culture.

STUDENTS FOR SENSIBLE DRUG POLICY
Founded: 1998

ssdp.org

One of the largest and fastest-growing student organizations on Earth, SSDP is the only international network of students dedicated to ending the war on drugs. They have chapters on more than 200 college and university campuses in the United States, and also play a leading role in statewide marijuana legalization campaigns and lobbying the federal government.

MARIJUANA POLICY PROJECT
Founded: 1995

mpp.org

A Washington, DC–based advocacy organization, MPP's mission is to "change federal law to allow states to determine their own marijuana policies without federal interference," while working to promote regulatory policies that treat marijuana no more harshly than alcohol. MPP has been a major force behind many successful medical marijuana and legalization initiatives, and typically uses Director of Communications Mason Tvert's "marijuana is safer than alcohol" messaging to frame the debate.

LAW ENFORCEMENT AGAINST PROHIBITION
Founded: 2002
leap.cc

Modeled after Vietnam Veterans Against the War, LEAP membership is open to those who actively fought the Drug War (police, prosecutors, judges, DEA agents) and now want to help end the destructive, racist, unconscionable War on Weed before any more lives are ruined. LEAP members actively work to replace prohibition with a system of legalization and regulation that will "end the violence, better protect human rights, safeguard our children, reduce crime and disease, treat drug abusers as patients, reduce addiction, use tax dollars more efficiently, and restore the public's respect and trust in law enforcement."

AMERICANS FOR SAFE ACCESS
Founded: 2002
safeaccessnow.org

The largest national organization focused solely on medical marijuana, ASA has more than 50,000 members around the world, and promotes the interests of medical-cannabis patients and providers by working to "resolve federal and state conflict on medical-cannabis laws, ensure safe and legal access to medical cannabis (therapy and research) throughout the nation, end stigma and discrimination associated with medical-cannabis use and research, and regulate cannabis like an herbal medicine."

WO/MEN'S ALLIANCE FOR
MEDICAL MARIJUANA
Founded: 1993
wamm.org

WAMM is the nation's oldest continuously operating medical-cannabis collective, one that still serves as a model of truly compassionate care. As you read on page 24, they've survived a DEA raid, handed out free medicine on the steps of city hall in Santa Cruz, California, and even successfully sued the federal government—all while servicing the seriously ill and those otherwise unable to afford medicine.

MARIJUANA MAJORITY
Founded: 2012
marijuanamajority.com

Marijuana Majority works "to help more people understand the simple fact that supporting commonsense solutions like regulating marijuana sales and ending marijuana arrests are mainstream positions and that there's no reason those who support reform should be afraid to say so." They provide a voice for commonsense cannabis policies in countless media stories while carefully compiling pro-legalization statements from celebrities, politicians, and opinion leaders as a way to reinforce the widespread support that already exists for ending pot prohibition.

DRUG POLICY ALLIANCE
Founded: 2000
drugpolicy.org

The nation's leading organization promoting drug policies that are grounded in science, compassion, health, and human rights, DPA serves as an umbrella group for many important efforts to both address the terrible consequences of drug prohibition and to change the policy itself. DPA is "actively involved in the legislative process and seeks to roll back the excesses of the drug war, block new, harmful initiatives, and promote sensible drug policy reforms," including by backing many successful statewide medical marijuana and full-legalization ballot initiatives.

MULTIDISCIPLINARY ASSOCIATION FOR PSYCHEDELIC STUDIES

Founded: 1986

maps.org

MAPS is a "non-profit research and educational organization that develops medical, legal, and cultural contexts for people to benefit from the careful uses of psychedelics and marijuana." They've been at the forefront of pushing the federal government to stop blocking vital research into the efficacy of whole-plant cannabis as a treatment for PTSD and other serious ailments.

POSTSCRIPT

Emily Post and her progeny have been the definitive source on etiquette for Americans since she first published her seminal guide *Etiquette* in 1922. Now in its eighteenth printing, the book maintains its cultural relevance nearly a century later by continuing to espouse an unshakable belief that while times do indeed change, good manners do not.

Personally, I couldn't agree more with that sentiment, particularly when it comes to smoking weed. Meanwhile, it turns out the Emily Post folks have been ahead of the curve on cannabis for a long time. Just check out how deftly the party-preparation section of their *Complete Book of Entertaining* handled the subject back in 1982:

> *Another problem that many hostesses face today is that of the guests who want to smoke marijuana. If the hostess approves of the practice and is untroubled by the fact that it is illegal, of course she has no problem. But if she does not approve and is concerned about people breaking the law in her home, she should say so firmly. The moment she sees the first joint being lighted or passed around she should tell her guests that she's sorry if she's being a spoilsport, but she doesn't want people smoking in her home where she would be held responsible if the illegal use of marijuana were detected. Then rather than letting the group continue to sit and chat, she should get some lively games or activities under way to distract them.*

Perfect advice with respect to all involved, including those who very rudely lit up in someone else's home without asking permission first (or at the very least inviting the hosts to join in). But what if this same scenario took place today, in one of the handful of places where smoking chronic is as legal as sipping Chablis?

🌿 PRO TIP 🌿

OVERGROW THE GOVERNMENT

"Even if one takes every reefer madness allegation of the prohibitionists at face value, marijuana prohibition has done far more harm to far more people than marijuana ever could."

—P. J. O'ROURKE, *BUSTED*

"Penalties against possession of a drug should not be more damaging to an individual than the use of the drug itself; and where they are, they should be changed. Nowhere is this more clear than in the laws against possession of marijuana in private for personal use."

—JIMMY CARTER, MESSAGE TO CONGRESS, 1977

To find out how legalization has (and hasn't) changed the rules when it comes to marijuana, I consulted Lizzie Post, great-granddaughter of Emily Post, author at the Emily Post Institute, and host of the *Awesome Etiquette* podcast. She confirmed plans to consider including a modern guide to marijuana in the upcoming nineteenth edition of *Etiquette,* and has already shared the following pot party advice with The Cannabist (the *Denver Post*'s marijuana-centric website).

1. HOST/HOSTESS GIFT: *Do you know for sure your host smokes pot? If they do, it's appropriate to bring as a gift. Remember: since it's a gift, your host doesn't have to smoke it with you, or even that night. A small glass jar or a pre-rolled joint or two makes for a classic presentation.*

2. KNOW YOUR AUDIENCE: *Is your new boss on the guest list? Is it dinner with your best friends? Whether as a guest or as a host, always be sure to ask permission and where your host would prefer you to smoke, just as you would with a cigarette.*

3. BRING YOUR OWN STASH: *Just like with alcohol, unless it's a gift, feel free to take your pot and glass with you when you leave.*

4. CHEF'S CHOICE: *Unlike wine, pot rarely messes up a menu. But never feel obligated to include it as part of the meal—or even the entire evening—if it's presented.*

5. R.E.S.P.E.C.T.: *Be respectful of those who don't smoke. Remember that even if the host is comfortable with it, some other guests might not be as pro-pot, so keep it casual and try not to let smoking turn into the main event for the night. While it may turn out that only a couple of you smoke, your offer should be to all guests at the party. Just the same way you wouldn't serve wine or dessert to only a couple guests, you should make sure there is enough pot for everyone to join in. Always be inclusive; sneaking off to smoke with just one or two other guests is not appropriate.*

Respect to you, Ms. Post. And consider this an open invitation to dinner next time you're in my neck of the woods.

. . . and please, RSVP.

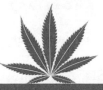

CHAPTER 4

Cannabis and Creativity

*When used properly, marijuana sparks
insight, innovation, and exhilaration.
By embracing, optimizing, and utilizing
that high, we can all lead healthier,
happier, more authentic lives.*

Despite the best propaganda efforts of the government, the media, and the pharmaceutical industry, the last five years have seen a growing recognition by the general public that marijuana is actually health-positive. Of course, the cannabis community has been making this claim for decades, based on direct experience, but until recently, ours were just voices in the wilderness.

Now, increasingly, the scientific community has finally begun to catch up, thanks to a veritable groundswell of major studies (mostly conducted outside the United States) confirming the plant's profound therapeutic benefits. And I believe that over the next five years, we'll see a similar revolution in our understanding of how marijuana positively affects mental health, again not just in treating conditions like depression, anxiety, PTSD, ADD, autism, and Alzheimer's, but also in sparking increased creativity, innovation, and overall happiness.

In 2010, for example, researchers from University College London published a paper entitled "Hyper-Priming in Cannabis Users: A Naturalistic Study of the Effects of Cannabis on Semantic Memory Function," which proved that smoking pot leads users to more quickly and efficiently mentally connect seemingly unrelated concepts—the exact kind of divergent thinking most associated with heightened imagination and innovation.

As *Wired* magazine reported:

> *A recent paper by scientists at University College, London looked at a phenomenon called semantic priming. This occurs when the activation of one word allows us to react more quickly to related words. . . .*
>
> *Interestingly, the scientists found that marijuana seems to induce a state of hyper-priming, in which the reach of semantic priming extends to distantly related concepts. As a result, we hear "dog" and think of nouns that, in more sober circumstances, would seem rather disconnected, such as "leash" or "hair." This state of hyper-priming helps explain why cannabis has been so often used as a creative fuel, as it seems to make the brain better at detecting those remote associations that lead to radically new ideas.*

So no, you don't just *feel* more creative when you're stoned. You *are* more creative, provided that you utilize your high.

In the popular consciousness, this type of cognitive enhancement is most often associated with artists, but perhaps only because they're freer to discuss the phenomenon than boldly innovative pot-smoking architects and accountants. And even then, no doubt we only hear from a small fraction of those who find cannabis an invaluable creative tool. In *Satchmo: My Life in New Orleans*, for example, jazz legend Louis Armstrong praised marijuana effusively as an invaluable "assistant" in his work of composing, performing, and improvising music, as well as a stalwart, lifelong friend. At least, he did in the original manuscript of the book, before his strong-arming, mob-tied manager cut out all positive mentions of pot prior to publication.

Of course, a few years later, when the same manager pressed Armstrong to pen a follow-up to his bestselling autobiography, the inventor of modern jazz rebuffed him by insisting he'd write another book only if the whole thing could be about *gage*—Satchmo's preferred slang term for marijuana. Armstrong then wrote a letter to President Dwight D. Eisenhower calling for total legalization of the herb. He also once tricked President Richard Nixon into carrying his weed-filled carry-on bag through security for him.

"If we all get as old as Methuselah, our memories will always be of lots of beauty and warmth from gage," Armstrong, who smoked three cigar-sized joints a day, told his friend Max Jones not long before he died. "Well, that was my life and I don't feel ashamed at all. Mary Warner, honey, you sure was good and I enjoyed you 'heap much.'"

So does that mean a budding young musician's money is better spent on a fat sack of weed than guitar lessons? Not hardly. But I would wager that there's more successful self-taught musicians on Earth than there are successful musicians who've never smoked pot.

🌿 PRO TIP 🌿
CANNABIS CHANGES
YOUR PERSPECTIVE

"I always have a joint, somewhere, near me, hidden. And I hardly touch it . . . but when I'm writing something—perfectly straight, perfectly sober—and I really pour it out, well, the next day, one hit of pot and it's 'punch up time.' And with that sort of judicious use, I find there's real value in it. Most of the things we use for creativity unfortunately don't always let you leave them alone, but pot does. And thank goodness for that."

—GEORGE CARLIN, *40 YEARS OF COMEDY*

"I should probably smoke more pot when I'm recording. You sit in the studio for four hours staring at a soundboard, and then you start to lose perspective. Smoking pot is a way of changing perspective."

—TREY ANASTASIO, *HIGH TIMES*

FREE YOUR MIND

When it comes to marijuana's mind-expanding capabilities, we tend to think of the Beatles having a laugh before working out a brilliant new song, or Hunter S. Thompson getting high while pounding away at his typewriter in a fit of mad genius, but it's not just "creative types" who benefit from the creativity boost of cannabis. Or, more accurately, every human being on Earth is the creative type, given the time and space to properly express that impulse. We all create language, behavior, art, and artifacts every single day, it's just that the default world of weed-hating squares teaches us to take it all for granted.

When really, who doesn't think we'd live in a nicer, happier, more just world if full-grown adults passed a joint and played freeze tag with strangers while waiting for the bus? But sadly that's just not how we've been socialized to live our lives. Play is for children, we're told, and art is for specialists. So instead we adhere to a crazy kind of false seriousness that nobody but fascists and assistant principals really believe in.

Which, at last, brings us to the real reason "the man" has always had it in for cannabis. Marijuana is one of the few mechanisms that can reliably subvert "Babylon System"—as Bob Marley dubbed consumerist capitalist culture—by revealing the utter absurdity of living in a wholly contrived world that values competition over compassion, strength over wisdom, greed over generosity, and conformity over novelty. As I've long said, pot's not antiestablishment because it's illegal, it's illegal because it's antiestablishment.

In other words, excessive imagination is a serious threat to the state, as it leads to imagining a better way to run the show than what the angry old men in charge now have got going. So yes, of course, the War on Weed is most certainly about protecting pharmaceutical companies, filling for-profit prisons, and keeping minorities down, but it's also about something much deeper, more fundamental. It's a war over the disputed territory that is your mind.

"Some people say marijuana is a crutch," comedian Doug Benson, host of *Getting Doug with High*, once observed. "Yeah, well, crutches *help* people walk. I think that's a good thing."

And so it is. But to truly smoke pot properly, you've got to transcend merely abiding in the world as it is, and get busy building a better world all your own. That means something different for every person, naturally, but I think if you sit down, alone, with a fat joint and a notepad—without worrying over the what-ifs and what-have-yous—you'll quickly get on to a few clues.

"Free your mind," as Parliament Funkadelic front man George Clinton so eloquently phrased it, "and your ass will follow."

Such freedom might lead your ass to form a psychedelic orchestra and rename yourself Dr. Funkenstein, or you might just decide to put down the damn phone for an hour, fill a bong with snow, and take a brisk walk around a frozen lake. Either way, the idea isn't to get stoned all the time but to *think* stoned all the time.

WHAT'S THE BIG *HIGH*-DEA?

If there's one thing leading neuroscientists and the writers of *Dude, Where's My Car?* share in common, it's a firm grasp of the fact that smoking pot can negatively affect short-term memory. Smoking pot can also negatively affect short-term memory.

Smoking pot *properly* therefore requires taking extra precautions against forgetfulness. So pick up a cheap reporter-style notebook that fits easily in your pocket and get used to using it extensively. Have one running list of everything you need to do (with subset lists devoted to the more complicated tasks), a list of things you're meaning to do (as opposed to things you *need* to do), and always blank pages in back for random "*high*-deas." Think of that section as the *back burner*, a place to let your more experimental marijuana epiphanies simmer for a while before either pouring them over rice or tossing them in the compost pile.

An example of a highdea I've had on the back burner for a

long time and still believe in would be bite-size bread bowls filled with chowder as a pass-around hors d'oeuvre. An example of a highdea I put on the back burner for a short period of time and then abandoned would be waterslides as a form of urban mass transit.

Anyway, while I wish I could take credit for coining the portmanteau "highdea," it's of unknown origins, even though Reddit has an official highdeas subreddit, and highdeas.com has more than 300,000 Facebook fans. Both also boast active online communities where users post their own stoned brainstorms and rate those of others.

According to highdeas.com's official definition, a highdea is "a unique idea or insight a person has while they are under the influence of cannabis that most likely would have not existed otherwise (like the one for this site)," which includes everything from the silly ("The word 'OK' looks like a sideways person"), to the profound ("What if Stephen Hawking's computer achieved sentience and was pretending to be a brilliant physicist to hide?"), to the profoundly silly ("If you watch *Jaws* backwards, it's a movie about a shark that keeps throwing up people until they have to open a beach.").

Sadly, without a notebook on constant call, all too many amazing highdeas escape, lost irretrievably in a haze of THC just minutes after they arrive. And don't ever discount the idea that the highdea that got away just might have been the best idea of your life. Consider what Carl Sagan had to say on the subject, writing an essay as "Mr. X" for *Marihuana Reconsidered*:

> *There is a myth about such highs: the user has an illusion of great insight, but it does not survive scrutiny in the morning. I am convinced that this is an error, and that the devastating insights achieved when high are real insights; the main problem is putting these insights in a form acceptable to the quite different self*

that we are when we're down the next day. Some of the hardest work I've ever done has been to put such insights down on tape or in writing. The problem is that ten even more interesting ideas or images have to be lost in the effort of recording one.

Take note that Sagan attributes marijuana-induced memory loss not to a mind full of neurons firing too slowly but rather one that's processing data much too quickly to keep it all straight (pun intended). Meanwhile, I firmly believe that despite all the technological advances of the modern era, there's still no quicker, more reliable way to get it all down than on paper. Also, unlike your phone, which is an incredibly powerful interactive distraction machine, a blank page just sits there waiting quietly until you write something. And it never runs low on batteries.

DANKS FOR THE MEMORIES

Let's be honest, if you've ever spent twenty stoned minutes looking for a pencil—just thirty seconds after you stopped using it—that's not always as hilarious a comedic proposal as Hollywood makes out. In fact, it's actually quite vexing. And it can really compromise the integrity of your high. (BTW: It was behind your ear the whole time!)

So here's some good news: By almost all accounts, marijuana's deleterious effect on memory seems to affect only short-term memory, and only while you're actually high. Which means put the blunt down, and before long you'll likely remember your iTunes password. Also, remember (ha!), while forgetfulness tends to get a bad rap, in most respects it's adaptive behavior. Just imagine trying to navigate a world where you remember *everything* you see, smell, hear, touch, and taste. How could you ever focus on breathing and swallowing, never mind lead a coherent, fulfilling life?

Which brings us to the *really* good news about marijuana and memory, namely that because of weed's special coevolutionary connection to our human minds, including a unique ability to engage the brain's natural endocannabinoid system and promote a state of homeostasis, the herb actually offers proven, profound neuroprotective benefits, whether you're struggling to remember or struggling to forget.

Let's start with those struggling to remember, since that's clearly the more counterintuitive cannabis indication. After all, if THC tends to impair short-term memory, why would you ever consider OG Kush to be good medicine for an Alzheimer's patient? The answer lies one paragraph above, in the word "homeostasis," or "the tendency toward a relatively stable equilibrium between interdependent elements, especially as maintained by physiological processes."

Basically, by keeping your mind on an even keel, the body's natural endocannabinoid system, when functioning properly, ensures that you remember and forget properly, among many other things. And if that functioning does go awry internally, ingesting cannabinoids derived from marijuana can help return the system to balance. Which means, all things considered, ganja's good for your brain. Again, not just in treating symptoms and conditions but also in actively protecting neurons from damage and disease.

At least, that's what the federal government claimed when

staking out Patent #6630507. Filed back in 1999, the patent—held by the US Department of Health and Human Services, and titled "Cannabinoids as neuroprotectants and antioxidants"—states definitively that compounds found in cannabis are "useful in the treatment and prophylaxis of a wide variety of oxidation associated diseases, such as ischemic, age-related, inflammatory and autoimmune diseases," and that the government has known this for more than fifteen years.

"Cannabinoids are found to have particular application as neuroprotectants," the patent reads, unequivocally. "For example in limiting neurological damage following . . . stroke and trauma, or in the treatment of neurodegenerative diseases, such as Alzheimer's disease, Parkinson's disease and HIV dementia."

Meanwhile, marijuana has also shown tremendous promise in treating post-traumatic stress disorder (PTSD), a debilitating condition that essentially stems from a persistent inability to "forget" a traumatic incident. PTSD affects untold millions of people around the world, and has led to an epidemic of suicides among America's combat veterans. And yet the very same government holding Patent #6630507 continues to block research into cannabis as a possible PTSD treatment.

FORGET WEED NOT

Getting high definitely fucks with your short-term memory, but follow these simple rules and even type-A neurotic herb smokers can learn to stop worrying and love the bong.

⚜ Put your keys and phone down in the exact same place every time you return home. Construct a small, colorful bin for them if it helps you get in the habit, as this alone will save you about two hours per week of anguish and heartache.

☙ Don't ever try to rush out the door when stoned, as you will forget something important and obvious without fail.

☙ Don't ever go food shopping when stoned, unless you've got an extensive, detailed shopping list and an iron will.

☙ Screen all calls when stoned. Ask yourself, "Would I want to talk to this person right now if they were sitting in front of me, or would I wish for a magic way to avoid talking to them without any social stigma?" Related: Don't stoned-dial anybody who doesn't already know you smoke weed.

☙ When I visited Hunter S. Thompson's former home and fortified compound in Woody Creek, Colorado, I was thrilled to find the walls still covered in notes he'd scrawled out and taped up all over the place, from shopping lists to enemy lists to love notes, publishing contracts, and inspirational aphorisms. I must have spent a solid hour reading them all like a kind of nonlinear journal. And then I promptly adopted the extremely useful system myself the minute I got home.

☙ When using cannabis while working on a creative project, get all the mundane and/or detail-oriented aspects of the initiative taken care of first, then get stoned and put your head to work on the more interesting stuff.

☙ Decide what you're going to do after you get stoned, before you get stoned. And then perhaps write it down and stick it on the wall.

THE ENHANCEMENT THEORY

Dr. Lester Grinspoon, associate professor emeritus at Harvard Medical School, began investigating marijuana in 1967 in an attempt to dissuade his best friend, famed astronomer Carl Sagan, from getting blazed all the time. But when he did a little digging down at the library to better make his case, Grinspoon instead discovered that he'd been duped. The government's case against marijuana was all based on "brainwashing and propaganda." So he offered Sagan a mea culpa, and then got to work writing his seminal 1971 book, *Marihuana Reconsidered*, in an attempt to set the record straight.

Sagan himself never spoke publicly about his abiding love of cannabis, but he did make his thoughts on the subject known to the universe by contributing an anonymous essay, writing:

> *I do not consider myself a religious person in the usual sense, but there is a religious aspect to some highs. The heightened sensitivity in all areas gives me a feeling of communion with my surroundings, both animate and inanimate. Sometimes a kind of existential perception of the absurd comes over me and I see with awful certainty the hypocrisies and posturing of myself and my fellow men. And at other times, there is a different sense of the absurd, a playful and whimsical awareness. Both of these senses of the absurd can be communicated, and some of the most rewarding highs I've had have been in sharing talk and perceptions and humor. Cannabis brings us an awareness that we spend a lifetime being trained to overlook and forget and put out of our minds.*

Sagan, writing as Mr. X, further praised marijuana's powers of cerebral expansion, including describing making a major breakthrough in understanding "the origins and invalidities of racism in terms of gaussian distribution curves" while "taking a shower with my wife while high." He then vigorously defended the validity of such pot-fueled epiphanies.

Clearly, he was a man who thought long and hard about how to utilize his high. And yet, despite being one of the most out-spoken, antiestablishment voices of his era, Sagan—out of un-derstandable fear for his career and family—only agreed to go on the record about these life-altering *eureka* moments posthu-mously. Which invites the question: *How many other celebrated intellects and innovators in history utilized cannabis's powers of cognitive enhancement to great acclaim without ever letting the rest of us in on their secret?*

A line of questioning that eventually led Dr. Grinspoon to theorize that pot's primary benefits include not only efficacy as a medicine and a recreational drug but also as a catalyst for creativity, and the enhancement of life's many splendors.

"Almost all of the research, writing, political activity, and legislation devoted to marijuana has so far been concerned only with the question of whether it is harmful and how much harm it does," Grinspoon observed. "The only exception is the grow-ing medical-marijuana movement, but as encouraging as that movement is, it still excludes marijuana's capacity to catalyze ideas and insights, heighten the appreciation of music and art, or deepen emotional and sexual intimacy. This property of 'enhancement' is therefore often misunderstood and under-appreciated—not only by non-users, but even by some users, especially young people mainly interested in promoting sociability and fun."

So to shed some light on this blind spot in the science, Dr. Grinspoon launched marijuana-uses.com, along with a call for people from all walks of life to contribute their own stories of how cannabis enhances their existence. And then he got the ball rolling personally, by sharing "To Smoke or Not to Smoke:

A Cannabis Odyssey"—a thoughtful, insightful reflection on his more than forty years as a physician, an academic, an author, and a leading marijuana-legalization advocate, which also includes a moving description of how medical marijuana helped ease the suffering of his son Danny, who died of leukemia at age fifteen.

> *On a normal day of chemotherapy, I hoped we could make it home from the hospital before Danny's vomiting would start, and we always had to put a big bucket next to his bed. But the first time he tried taking a few puffs prior to a round of treatments, he got off the gurney and said, "Mom, there's a sub shop in Brookline. Could we stop for a sub-sandwich on the way home?" And all I thought was, "Wow."*

By allowing certain of his colleagues to witness this phenomenon firsthand, Dr. Grinspoon eventually convinced the head of the oncology department at Boston Children's Hospital to undertake a 1975 study, published in *The New England Journal of Medicine*, that for the first time demonstrated the efficacy of cannabinoids for nausea and vomiting associated with chemotherapy. But ironically, the more he came to appreciate the plant's unique healing properties, and came to be known as the guy who'd literally written the book on marijuana, the more strenuously Dr. Grinspoon resisted the urge to light up himself—despite a lot of urging from Carl Sagan. As he explained when I interviewed him for VICE's technology vertical, *Motherboard*:

> *As I researched and wrote* Marihuana Reconsidered, *I knew I wanted to have this experience, but I also knew that if the book was successful, I'd be called upon to appear before committees and testify in court, and I didn't want to compromise my posi-*

*tion. In other words, I didn't want this to become a N-of-1
study. I wanted to be as objective as possible. So I waited.*

Dr. Grinspoon held out for about two years before realizing
that he'd never truly understand marijuana without experimenting a bit on himself. He would rather famously go on to become
a devoted and enthusiastic herbalist, but his very first attempt at
getting high proved to be "the only negative experience" he ever
had with cannabis, as he explained in the same essay:

Ever since Marihuana Reconsidered *came out people had been
asking me: "Wait, you wrote a book about marijuana and
you've never tried it?" And I'd reply, "Well, I wrote a book
about schizophrenia too, and I haven't tried that!"*

*But then [my wife Betsy and I] went to a party and smoked
until everyone else in the circle, including Carl, waved it off.
They were all apparently stoned, while Betsy and I felt nothing.
At which point, I began to get very anxious—could I have written a book about a grand placebo?*

*When I got home, I couldn't sleep. Betsy had to remind me
that my own research revealed many people don't get high the
first time they smoke. Carl, in his Mr. X essay, said he'd had to
try something like six times to experience a high. So the next
weekend we smoked again, and it still didn't work. But then the
third time, I remember after the joint Betsy and I were standing
around with another couple in the kitchen, eating a napoleon—
the four of us passing it around. And you know that viscous
material between the layers? It kept sliding back and forth,
threatening to fall on the floor. We were having a hilarious time!*

*So Betsy asked, "Where did you get this napoleon, it's
unbelievably good. We've never had anything like it." And
when they named the bakery, we were surprised to discover
we'd eaten their napoleons before!*

Meanwhile, Sgt. Pepper's Lonely Hearts Club Band *was on the hi-fi, a record I'd actually heard before many times. My son David would put it on and say, "Dad, you ought to get your head out of the Baroque and listen to the Beatles." But I didn't see the appeal. Until that night, under the influence of marijuana, when I heard the Beatles for the first time. And it was like an auditory implosion. I couldn't believe it!*

And so the enhancement theory was born.

Interesting postscript: About a year later, Dr. Grinspoon would have a chance to relate that *Sgt. Pepper's* experience directly to John Lennon, over dinner, the night before the former Beatle's 1975 deportation hearing in front of the Immigration and Naturalization Service. Grinspoon had agreed to testify as an expert witness at the hearing, after the Nixon administration—which took a decidedly dim view of Lennon's recent anti–Vietnam War activities—dug up an old hashish bust in London as an excuse to kick him out of the country.

As recounted in "To Smoke or Not to Smoke":

I told John how cannabis appeared to make it possible for me to "hear" his music for the first time in much the same way that Allen Ginsberg reported that he had "seen" Cézanne for the first time when he purposely smoked cannabis before setting out for the Museum of Modern Art. John was quick to reply that I had experienced only one facet of what marijuana could do for music, that he thought it could be very helpful for composing and making music as well as listening to it.

In many ways, that dinner epitomizes everything we've been talking about in this book. On one side of the table, we have a formerly angry, alienated young man who experienced a creative and spiritual awakening the first time he tried cannabis (with Bob Dylan!), a transformation that profoundly enhanced not just his art, but his life. Marijuana also helped him see through the lies of the government, so he started speaking out against war and injustice, only to have the government turn around and use marijuana as a thinly veiled excuse to threaten his freedom.

And across from John Lennon, we have a medical doctor and Harvard professor who, despite all his education, training, and experience, blindly believed the government's lies about marijuana, until his best bud (Carl Sagan!) sent him running to the medical library, where he discovered through data what so many of us learned through direct experience—that's there's absolutely no basis for marijuana prohibition. Next, the very same plant revealed its profound healing powers via his son, leading to research that subsequently brought relief to untold millions, who learned for the first time, with scientific certainty, that cannabis helps ease the pain and nausea of chemo treatments. And then marijuana at last opened Dr. Grinspoon himself up to the music of the very man he'd later travel to New York City to meet and help defend from the government.

Telling the story at the 2011 national NORML conference, where he accepted a Lifetime Achievement Award, Dr. Grinspoon recalled that John Lennon's original London arrest had been engineered by a notorious Scotland Yard sergeant who specialized in busting rock musicians for drugs. Lennon claimed that while he certainly smoked hashish at the time, the drugs used to make the case were planted.

Fortunately, the next day, in the case of *United States v. John Lennon*, thanks to some quick thinking by Dr. Grinspoon, justice prevailed.

I was on the witness stand and the federal prosecutor asked me, "Well, now, as you know, Mister Lennon was convicted on hashish charges and since the law in the United States doesn't mention hashish, just marijuana, Dr. Grinspoon, let's clear up the first fact, that hashish and marijuana are indeed the same thing. Aren't they?"

And I said, "No."

I have to admit I felt compromised a little bit because if I was to behave like a pure scientist, I might have said, "Well, they're different but here are the things that they have in common . . ." But I just said no, and figured, "Hey, if the government wants to bring out the close relationship between marijuana and hashish they're gonna have to fish for it. I'm not going to do their work for them.

So I was astonished when the prosecutor said, "They are not the same?"

He was dumbfounded, as that was his whole case.

The prosecutor then went to the judge, they conferred, and this went on for some time. Until finally the judge said the government has dropped its case and we walked out of the courtroom.

IS MARIJUANA AN APHRODISIAC?

Thousands of years ago, the earliest tantric practitioners ceremonially consumed powerfully psychoactive doses of THC via a sacred edible called *bhang*, then sought to achieve total enlightenment by tapping into the body's deepest sexual energy through intense rituals that combined fasting, chanting, yoga, incense, and intercourse.

Sounds like a good deal all around, but those seeking a bit more "hard science" before committing to giving stoned sex a whirl probably shouldn't hold their breath. Because if the federal government steadfastly blocks research into marijuana as a treatment for severe PTSD in combat veterans on the grounds that the herb's just too dangerous to put in the hands of former marines, commandoes, and tank commanders, what are the chances they're going to supply researchers seeking an all-natural aphrodisiac?

Meanwhile, when a 2010 article in *Psychology Today* looked at what limited data does exist, the magazine determined that "the sexual effects of every other mood-altering drug—alcohol, amphetamines, antidepressants, cocaine, narcotics—are well-documented, fairly consistent, and not particularly controversial . . . [but] oddly, marijuana's sexual effects are highly unpredictable, from strongly sex-inhibiting to strongly sex-enhancing."

So what accounts for that wide gap? Set and setting, plus opportunity, dosage, biochemistry, and, perhaps most significantly, the user's own intentions. For a VICE *Motherboard* article exploring the subject, I spoke with leading "sexpert" and enthusiastic pot smoker Susie Bright, who confirmed that one size indeed does not fit all when it comes to mixing ganja and getting it on.

"If you have a party and everybody smokes pot, there's going be a couple of people who turn inward, and don't feel sexy," she told me. "Others will feel flirtatious, and open to suggestion. So it's hard to identify universal truths when it comes to cannabis and pleasure."

The same individual may also react much differently to marijuana in different contexts, according to Bright, best known for cofounding *On Our Backs*, the world's first women's sex magazine, and serving as one of America's founding sex-positive feminists. Now the host of a popular podcast, she explains that in her vast experience—including one highly memorable "pot-brownie orgy"—cannabis works best as an aphrodisiac in small-to-moderate doses. Otherwise, you risk getting sluggish, or slipping into introspective "navel gazing."

She also offered a helpful suggestion for avoiding those potholes: "Whenever someone asks, 'What's the greatest drug combo for sex?' I always reply, 'cannabis and espresso.'"

SIX RULES FOR SEXIER STONED SEX

1. Do not attempt to lose your pot virginity and your actual virginity simultaneously. Instead, smoke pot and have sex separately first—sufficiently to achieve basic competence in both—before attempting to combine the two.

2. Always have plenty of refreshing nonalcoholic beverages on hand, as cottonmouth is a huge turn-off. Also, nothing beats some nice dark chocolate to tingle the taste buds, and give your high an extra little kick.

3. Experiment with lower doses of THC—just enough to enhance your sensory perceptions—before attempting to fuck while high as fuck.

4. In moderation, edibles make for an ideal aphrodisiac, as they offer a powerful body buzz that comes on slowly, builds to an intense peak, and then gently tails off over the course of a few hours. But eat too much weed-laced biscotti and you might end up struggling just to get your shoes off, never mind go all the way.

5. Ideally, smoke a *sativa* strain prior to making love for a quick jolt of erotic energy, and then an *indica* when the deed's done, to enhance the warm fuzzies. Some anecdotal evidence also indicates that high-CBD strains improve sexual performance.

6. If one partner enjoys cannabis and the other doesn't, don't ever let it become a cause for shaming or cajoling.

HIGH CULTURE THROUGH THE AGES

From the invention of jazz to the birth of hip-hop, from the Club des Hashischins of Dumas, Balzac, Hugo, and Baudelaire to the beatnik crash pads of Kerouac, Burroughs, Cassady, and Ginsberg, cannabis has helped inspire and elevate some of history's most transformative cultural movements. So here's a chronic chronology of just a few of the weed-fueled art scenes that shaped the modern world.

Congo Square (New Orleans, Early 1800s)

The seeds of America's counterculture first sprouted in the early 1800s in New Orleans's Congo Square, where on Sundays the local black population, including many slaves, gathered for ritualized drumming, dancing, and an outdoor market that blended African traditions with elements of the city's American, European, Caribbean, and Creole culture. Eventually, local whites and even visitors from foreign lands started making pilgrimages to witness the exotic goings-on (which included copious marijuana smoking)—at least until the increasingly popular assemblages were banned by the city in 1843. At that point, the powerful musical energy originating in Congo Square splintered off in different directions, pushing the black Christian churches of the South toward what became Gospel music, while also giving rise to a decidedly secular jazz scene that felt far more at home among the city's prostitutes, gamblers, pimps, players, and vipers than in any church.

As jazz evolved from a spontaneous counterculture ritual into America's most popular musical genre, reefer-friendly jazz musicians began to tour, leaving a trail of newly initiated marijuana smokers (and freshly planted marijuana seeds) in their wake while crisscrossing the country to perform. Many cited marijuana as a positive influence not only on their playing but also on their lives and communities—particularly when compared to alcohol. So it's not surprising that a wide range of jazz greats made approving references to reefer, gage, muggles, Mary Jane, and other slang for the herb in their songs.

For a real kick, I highly recommend picking up one of the better compilation albums that collect these old "reefer songs" from the 1930s and '40s. You'll encounter some of the biggest names of the era at their stoniest best on tracks like "Reefer Man" (Cab Calloway), "Texas Tea Party" (Benny Goodman), "Muggles" (Louis Armstrong), "Gimme a Pigfoot (Gimme a Reefer)" (Bessie Smith), "When I Get Low, I Get High" (Ella Fitzgerald), and "I'm Feeling High and Happy" (Gene Krupa).

The Club des Hashischins (Paris, Mid-1800s)

The French first began consuming hashish in 1789, when soldiers tasked by Napoleon with invading Egypt picked up the local custom and brought it home with them after the campaign. By the mid-1800s, despite a pervasive government prohibition, some of the age's brightest minds were nonetheless meeting secretly in Paris, for cannabis-spiked coffee, as part of the legendary Club des Hashischins, including Alexandre Dumas, Victor Hugo, Honoré de Balzac, and Charles Baudelaire.

"It was in an old house on the Île St-Louis, the Pimodan hotel built by Lauzun, where the strange club which I had recently joined held its monthly séance," philosopher, author, and journalist Théophile Gautier wrote of his first visit to the Club des Hashischins in the literary journal *Revue des Deux Mondes*. "The doctor stood by a buffet on which lay a platter filled with small Japanese saucers. He spooned a morsel of paste or greenish jam about as large as a thumb from a crystal vase, and placed it next to the silver spoon on each saucer. The doctor's face radiated enthusiasm; his eyes glittered, his purple cheeks were aglow, the veins in his temples stood out strongly, and he breathed heavily through dilated nostrils. 'This will be deducted from your share in Paradise,' he said as he handed me my portion...."

The doctor was Jacques-Joseph Moreau, a leading psychiatrist of the day, whose personal experiments with hashish inspired him to pioneer the study of how drugs affect the central nervous system. The Club des Hashischins basically served as Dr. Moreau's stoned guinea pigs—a group of highly cerebral, extremely articulate test subjects to observe in close quarters as they consumed hashish in precisely measured amounts, which, according to various members' accounts of the experience, proved strong enough to bring on celestial voices, divine visions, and powerful hallucinations. One can only imagine the effect these sessions had on their art—and lives.

The Beats (New York City, Late 1940s)

Amid the stifling cultural conformity that followed World War II, the Greatest Generation drank heavily and smoked endless cigarettes—as Hollywood and Madison Avenue taught them to—while almost universally eschewing marijuana as an agent of addiction, subversion, and death.

Fortunately, certain among their children, who'd come of age on the reefer-fueled jazz of Louis Armstrong and Cab Calloway, roundly rejected the square world's fast-spinning hamster wheel of conspicuous consumerism in favor of a bold new kind of bohemianism that blended the improvisational jazz and free-verse poetry happening in Harlem with the radical politics and avant-garde art scene of Greenwich Village, plus a little Eastern mysticism and plenty of grass rolled into the mix.

Eventually this so-called Beat Generation would grow to global influence, including as "*roll* models" for the later San Francisco hippie scene, but it started among a small group of highly literate, dissident, somewhat depraved students and hangers-on at New York's Columbia University, a cannabis-friendly crew that included Jack Kerouac, Allen Ginsberg, Neal Cassady, and William S. Burroughs. In his authoritative social history of marijuana, *Smoke Signals*, author Martin Lee beautifully described how these young writers and poets learned to utilize their high:

> *Kerouac and his cohorts got high together in small groups, much like the bohemian writers who congregated at the Hashish Eaters' Club in mid-nineteenth-century Paris. The Beats were conscious of their link to this great stoned lineage of European artists, which included the Dadaists, Surrealists, Symbolists, and others who defied convention and labels. Kerouac's cabal loved the associational fluidity engendered by cannabis, how it loosened the powers of analogy and unleashed the spoken word. They stayed up all night smoking fat marijuana bombers, listening to jazz, reciting poetry, and confiding their deepest secrets, their hopes and fears, in protracted, stoned rap sessions.*
>
> *As Beat poet Allen Ginsberg recalled: "All that we knew was*

*that we were making sense to each other, you know talking from
heart to heart, and that everybody else around us was talking
like some kind of strange, lunar robots in business suits."*

The Provos (Amsterdam, Early 1960s)

We all know Amsterdam is a haven for cannabis freedom and
is one of the most bicycle-friendly cities on Earth. But few realize that what both of those progressive public policies (and
many others) have in common is the Dutch Provo movement,
which pre-dated the hippies, the Yippies, and the New Left in
its use of confrontational street performance, subversive art, and
impromptu political demonstrations—all designed to under-
mine a system run by "despicable plastic people," in the words
of Provo founding father Robert Jasper Grootveld.

A master of using outrageous publicity stunts to garner press
coverage and galvanize public support, Grootveld served as
court jester for an absurdist movement with serious ideas about
police reform, economic injustice, and social liberation. For example, to prove the authorities' total ignorance regarding marijuana, and thus the total illegitimacy of their prohibition against
it, Grootveld and his fellow Provos created "Marihuettegame,"
which consisted of repeatedly baiting the police into arresting
them for something that looked like marijuana but was actually
another herb.

Led by anarchistic young radicals, artists, and academics,
the Provos—through their writing, music, and chaotic
"happenings"—pushed the government into making bicycling a
priority and tolerating the cannabis coffeeshops. Eventually,
their ongoing clashes with the law led to the dismissal of Amsterdam's authoritarian police chief and the resignation of the mayor.
The city's been a beacon of freedom and tolerance ever since.

🌿 PRO TIP 🌿
EMBRACE CANNABIS CULTURE

"Like others, I spent a lot of time in jazz clubs, nursing the two-beer minimum. I put on hornrimmed sunglasses at night. I went to parties in lofts where girls wore strange attire. I was hugely tickled by all forms of marijuana humor, though the talk back then was in inverse relation to the availability of that useful substance."

—THOMAS PYNCHON, *SLOW LEARNER*

Haight-Ashbury (San Francisco, Mid-1960s)

Smoking pot was so integral to the psychedelic music and art movement that emerged in San Francisco in the late 1960s that even today the most common horrible hackneyed lede for a story about marijuana remains: *Once exclusively the purview of Jerry Garcia and the flower children of the '60s, today Mary Jane's all grown up—into a multibillion-dollar legal industry . . .*

Still, it is sort of mind-blowing to think that the Grateful Dead, Jefferson Airplane, Janis Joplin, and Jimi Hendrix once lived within blocks of one another. In a 1967 article for the *New York Times Magazine* titled "The Hashbury Is the Capital of the Hippies," a still relatively unknown Hunter S. Thompson described this famed Haight-Ashbury neighborhood, which he also then called home, as "the orgiastic tip of a great psyche-delic iceberg."

"Marijuana is everywhere," Thompson wrote of his beloved Hashbury. "People smoke it on the sidewalks, in doughnut shops, sitting in parked cars or lounging on the grass in Golden

Gate Park. . . . The only way to write honestly about the scene is to be part of it, yet to write from experience is an admission of felonious guilt; it is also a potential betrayal of people whose only 'crime' is the smoking of a weed that grows wild all over the world but the possession of which, in California, carries a minimum sentence of two years in prison for a second offense and a minimum of five years for a third. So, despite the fact that the whole journalism industry is full of unregenerate heads—just as many journalists were hard drinkers during Prohibition—it is not very likely that the frank, documented truth about the psychedelic underworld, for good or ill, will be illuminated at any time soon in the public prints."

Things started to head south just a few months later, when the Grateful Dead were set up for a marijuana bust at their communal Hashbury home. In fact, that kind of heavy police repression, along with a huge influx of tourist gawkers and sleazy opportunists, soon broke up the scene, but Jerry Garcia, for one, never lost his fondness for Mary Jane.

"To get really high is to forget yourself," Captain Trips told *Rolling Stone* in 1972, "and to forget yourself is to see everything else—and to see everything else is to become an understanding molecule in evolution, a conscious tool of the universe. And I think every human being should be a conscious tool of the universe. That's why I think it's important to get high."

The Outlaws (Nashville, Tennessee, Late 1960s)

Imagine a smoke-filled recording studio and rehearsal space in Nashville, Tennessee, in the late 1960s, where a group of young, relatively unknown musicians gather to pass a few joints around and discuss their growing disillusionment with the increasingly mainstream pop ethos that's steadily taking over country music. Although they made a living in those days as songwriters, session players, and sidemen by sticking to the formulaic "Nashville Sound" that the recording industry demanded, the radio expected, and audiences had grown used to, Willie Nelson, Kris Kristofferson, Waylon Jennings, and their weed-friendly contemporaries all pined to play a much grittier, rawer, more emotionally honest style that hearkened back to country's days as the music of roadhouses and honky-tonks.

The first of their breed to hit the big time with a rough-and-tumble image had been Johnny Cash, whose habit of writing and performing hit songs while breaking all the rules eventually paved the way for what came to be called Outlaw Country. Soon the most popular male singers in the South wore denim and leather, grew their hair long, sported facial hair, and smoked cigarettes that looked funny and didn't smell like a Marlboro.

"You may be high," reads the popular Internet meme, "but you'll never be Johnny Cash eating cake in a bush high."

The photo the meme accompanies and describes, by the way, comes from the back cover of Cash's 1976 album *Strawberry Cake*, so it's not like he was exactly embarrassed about being caught in flagrante with an entire cake while stoned to the gills and sitting in the dirt. Cash also stood up for the herb, and free speech, in 1970, while working on *The Johnny Cash Show* on ABC television. When network producers objected to the lyrics of Kris Kristofferson's hit song "Sunday Morning, Coming Down" and demanded that he change the line, "I'm wishing Lord that I was stoned," the Man in Black took on the suits and performed his friend's single as it was written.

In time, of course, Willie Nelson would become an American icon while remaining almost synonymous with marijuana in the public imagination. And if you think "American icon" and "almost synonymous with marijuana" is overstating the case, kindly name me another beloved public figure who has proudly copped to smoking weed on the roof of the White

House, as Nelson did in his 1988 autobiography *Willie*. "Sitting on the roof of the White House in Washington, DC, late at night with a beer in one hand and a fat Austin Torpedo in the other," he recalled. "I let the weed cover me with a pleasing cloud. . . . I guess the roof of the White House is the safest place to smoke dope."

So does the redheaded stranger, who's been arrested four times for pot possession, remain an outlaw to this day? Well, here's what he told *Rolling Stone* magazine in 2014, at age eighty-one: "[The police] don't really bother me anymore for weed, because you can bust me now and I'll pay my fine or go to jail, get out and burn one on the way home. They know they're not stopping me."

Trenchtown (Jamaica, Early 1970s)

Adherents of Jamaica's Rastafarian movement cultivated and consumed cannabis as part of their religious practice—including before and during drumming and chanting sessions—for more than four decades before the first reggae songs started sprouting up in 1967. Rastas smoke ganja as a sacrament to cleanse the body and mind, and believe it helps them commune with God, while rejecting the materialism and oppression of Babylon in favor of a life devoted to spiritual authenticity. Referencing Revelation 22:2, they often refer to the herb as "the healing of the nations."

Originally, the Rasta movement largely kept to Jamaica's rugged backcountry, but around the time Bob Marley came of age, the religion began to take root among the poor, disaffected youth in Kingston, the island's capital city, including the rough-and-tumble Trenchtown neighborhood Marley called home. In 1966, at age twenty-one, the aspiring young musician officially joined the faith, as did many other popular reggae artists in

Jamaica, who would later collectively help transform the Caribbean island's vibrant music scene from a local treasure into an herb-fueled international sensation.

Along with Jimmy Cliff, Desmond Dekker, Lee "Scratch" Perry, Peter Tosh, Bunny Wailer, and countless others, Marley developed his music and his message by working with incredibly talented local musicians and fellow spiritual seekers, who often came together to smoke ganja, play instruments, and share stories. Thanks to these artists, reggae music would become a powerful global soundtrack of resistance—including standing up for your right to smoke herb—with Bob Marley himself making his feelings clear on tracks like "Rebel Music (3 O'Clock Roadblock)," "Kaya," "African Herbsman," and "Three Little Birds."

Kalakuta Republic (Nigeria, 1970s)

In his signature song "Expensive Shit," Afro-beat founding father and legendary herbsman Fela Kuti recounts one of the more unusual criminal cases in the history of marijuana prohibition. Kuti had enraged the government of Nigeria by, among other things, criticizing the country's corrupt military and political leaders, openly smoking cannabis, rejecting monotheistic religion, marrying twenty-seven different women in one day, and, eventually, building his own compound, declaring it the fully independent Kalakuta Republic, and running it as a freak-fest-commune cum recording studio/nightclub.

In retaliation, the authorities decided to set up Africa's most celebrated musician for a marijuana bust, just like what had happened to John Lennon in England a decade earlier—only Kuti managed to discover and eat the planted joint before the police had time to find the evidence. Not to be discouraged, however, the cops hauled him in anyway, determined to wait for their prisoner to take an expensive shit they could then use to incriminate him. From there, the story gets a bit, shall we say, *murky*, but legend has it that the pot-loving polygamist triumphed by borrowing the feces of a fellow inmate and claiming them as his own.

In any event, Fela Kuti remained an outspoken proponent of cannabis throughout his life, to the extent that he not only allowed the musicians in his band to consume large amounts of ganja before performing, he often required they do so. And despite his rather eccentric personality, there must have been some method to his madness, because he became one of the most popular and influential musicians of the 1970s by blending traditional African percussion and rhythms with jazz, funk, soul, and rock music.

"Marijuana is my best friend because it is a gift of the creator to Africans," Kuti once said. "Marijuana has five fingers of creation . . . it enhances all your five senses."

Boogie-Down Bronx (New York City, Late 1970s)

In 2011, at the twenty-third annual *High Times* Cannabis Cup in Amsterdam, I had the distinct pleasure of standing backstage and burning a fat joint of Sativa Cup–winning Moonshine Haze while watching Coke La Rock and Busy Bee get inducted into the Counterculture Hall of Fame, an honor the magazine bestows upon cultural figures who've played a leading role in bringing true cannabis consciousness to the world.

Today, of course, hip-hop is a global phenomenon, one that Madison Avenue has long learned how to cash in on. But back in the day, the movement started as a spontaneous artistic uprising in the parks and on the streets of the Bronx, where young

DJs, MCs, break dancers, and graffiti artists used music, dance, and guerrilla murals to make their voices heard amid the din of the city's most beat-down borough.

In the late 1970s, Coke La Rock and Busy Bee were among the first MCs to perform regularly, using a microphone to amplify their often-improvised vocals to the sounds of a DJ spinning records. And not coincidentally, they also shared a day job back then—as marijuana dealers—that helped them make ends meet while perfecting their craft and finding an audience.

I hung around those two true OGs of the rap game for a bit during their time in Amsterdam, and found they spent as much time reminiscing about the various weed spots they used to frequent, and who had New York City's best herb supply back in those days, as they did marveling at how far things have progressed since being the biggest MC in hip-hop meant performing at your friend's sister's birthday party for pocket change and a few joints.

Techno Utopia (Goa, India, Mid-1980s)

A small state in Western India with miles of picturesque beaches on the Arabian Sea, incredible architecture, and a lush local environment awash in tropical flora and fauna, Goa has been luring spiritual seekers to its shores for at least 20,000 years, as evidenced by rock art engravings on the river Kushavati that provide the earliest evidence of human life in India.

In the late 1960s, international hippies began flocking to Goa, in search of a place to blend ancient mystical wisdom and New Age grooviness, while puffing the highest quality *charas* (hashish) on Earth—readily available at incredibly reasonable prices.

By the 1980s, inspired by the vibrant local ecstatic dance

scene and the increasing popularity of electronic music worldwide, foreign DJs and Indian musicians began collaborating on a style of electronica that came to be known as Goa trance. Over many smoky sessions, travelers played electronic music brought in on tape from all over the globe for "Goan heads," who incorporated those sounds into their scene's distinctive blend of psychedelic rock and some of the trippiest traditional music known to man.

The results turned on the revelers at Goa's now legendary full-moon raves, and from there literally spread around the world, helping to kick-start an EDM movement that's still fueled by weed, beats, and musical cross-pollination today.

ROOT-LEVEL INNOVATION: WHEN HIGH TECH GETS HIGH

"The best way I would describe the effect of the marijuana and the hashish is that it would make me relaxed and creative."

That's what Steve Jobs told an interrogator from the Department of Defense, in 1988, during a two-hour interview to determine if the famously tight-lipped technology mogul could qualify for a top-secret security clearance. At the time, the visionary genius behind Apple computers had just helped develop a cutting-edge imaging computer, and the military wanted access to it for use in airborne reconnaissance missions—however, a standard background check revealed Jobs's predilection for getting high.

In the end, despite his pot-smoking past and lack of remorse for same, Jobs got his security clearance. At the time, the Reagan administration was publicly equating marijuana use with murder, insanity, treason, and worse, but why let *that* get in the way of America's strategic interests? And just in case you think boldly creative tech types have stopped smoking weed since then, or the feds have gotten any less hypocritical about it, check out what James Comey, head of the FBI, recently told the *Wall Street Journal*, by way of explaining why a hiring ban against anyone who'd used marijuana in the last three years was preventing him from effectively staffing the bureau's anti-cybercrime division.

"One of my challenges is—I've got to hire a great workforce to keep pace with the criminals, and I am competing with a lot of better paying private sector entities for these kids," Comey said. "And some of those kids want to smoke weed on the way to their interview with the FBI."

It's funny because it's true.

Seriously though, you've sort of got to feel for FBI Director Comey's predicament. Trying to assemble a team of top-level computer hackers to defend against cyber terrorists without in-cluding ganja smokers is a lot like trying to form a reggae band without including ganja smokers: technically possible, but seriously ill advised.

RUSH JOB

In 2012, I got to interview Rush guitarist Alex Lifeson for *High Times* based on a referral from our mutual friends the Trailer Park Boys. (Alex made a hilarious cameo appearance in per-haps the best-loved episode of the cult classic Canadian TV series, and I'm in season 7, episode 3, for five seconds as "Greasy Stoner #1.")

Anyway, based on that rather shaky connection, Lifeson

greeted me on the roof deck of a luxury hotel in downtown Los Angeles while in town to finish up recording Rush's twenty-first studio album, *Clockwork Angels*. And despite being part of one of rock's truly chart-topping acts—a power trio, second only to the Beatles and the Rolling Stones for the most consecutive gold or platinum albums—he couldn't have been more gracious or accommodating.

When I asked him my favorite interview question—if cannabis plays a role in his creative process—he confirmed that Mary Jane can indeed prove a powerful muse, but only when used properly.

"I find that I can be very imaginative when stoned, very creative—but implementation is sometimes difficult," he responded. "In the very, very early days, occasionally—well, more than 'occasionally'—[drummer] Neil [Peart] and I would smoke a joint before going on. I mean, this is in the mid-'70s; I would never, ever do something like that now. I won't even have a sip of beer before a show, because I need to be extremely clearheaded. Of course, some people can smoke and remain clearheaded—just not me. But when we were younger and a little crazier, and were only playing for 25 minutes to a small crowd, it was okay to smoke before a show. I still played well."

To adapt an already apocryphal Hemingway aphorism, Lifeson seems to be saying: *Write stoned; perform sober.*

But that's just one person's experience, and your mileage may vary. It certainly wouldn't be difficult to put together an all-star band of musicians with no problem rocking while high. So definitely take the time to "experiment with marijuana" on your own until you discover how it best serves your creative process.

Just don't ever forget that cannabis is meant to be an aid to creativity, not a substitute.

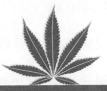

CHAPTER 5

The New Green Economy

*Experts predict the legal cannabis
industry will reach $8 billion in annual
sales (or higher!) in the next few years.
So what better way to "follow your
bliss" than by working in this exciting,
rewarding, rapidly growing field?*

From the moment Colorado and Washington became the first states to legalize marijuana in 2012, the corporate media has consistently framed the issue to the One Percent's liking by focusing myopically on the "green rush" aspect of things, via a steady stream of special reports on how "a new breed" of well-pedigreed professionals has come riding in like the cavalry to "legitimize" marijuana and reap huge profits in the process. Just think about how many cable news shows you've seen breathlessly reporting on the upside potential of the legal cannabis business ("Marijuana, Inc." "The Pot Barons," "The Cannabis Boom," "High Profits," etc.) versus those tallying up the social-justice and human-rights gains made since legalization.

Heck, even the herb's organized opponents have picked up on this shiny new media obsession, such as Kevin Sabet, co-founder of Smart Approaches to Marijuana, director of the Drug Policy Institute at the University of Florida, former senior adviser at the White House Office of National Drug Control Policy, human paraquat, and mouthpiece of a pretty much indefensible policy, who now makes opposition to "Big Marijuana" his main talking point when it comes to shouting down legalization.

"Remember Big Tobacco? Say hello to Big Marijuana," he opines in a typical blog post. "That's what we're about to get if we continue to legalize marijuana here in the United States. . . . Legalization is all about the mighty dollar—the money to be made by big marijuana businesses. . . . Indeed, we are ushering in a massive, profit-hungry industry, promoting addiction by commercializing and marketing the drug to our most vulnerable."

Which invites a few questions of Mr. Sabet, like: Since tobacco is highly addictive and kills 5 million people every year (Centers for Disease Control and Prevention), while cannabis has never killed anyone in 10,000 years of human consumption, do you support dismantling Big Tobacco by making cigarettes illegal? If so, what do you imagine will replace Philip Morris once tobacco goes into the black market? And if not, how can you justify allowing tobacco and outlawing marijuana?

And that just covers the surface hypocrisy. The real logical fallacy in Sabet's rhetorical gambit is that anyone who gives the matter more than a moment's thought soon comes to realize that Big Marijuana already exists, as Bill Piper, director of national affairs for the pro-legalization advocacy organization the Drug Policy Alliance made sure to point out during a debate with Sabet at the National Press Club.

"We already have 'Big Marijuana'—they're called drug cartels, and they chop people's heads off," Piper noted rather sharply. "So why let these thugs keep billions of dollars a year if we don't have to?"

Still, while I don't give Kevin Sabet credit for anything beyond opportunism, I too have some serious concerns about Big Marijuana. Because when it comes to "legitimizing" the herb, I happen to think that Corporate America has a lot more to learn from cannabis culture than the other way around.

I began exploring that thesis in 2013 with my first ever VICE feature, titled "Get Rich or High Trying: The Coming Age of Corporate Cannabis." In it, I spoke with Brendan Kennedy, a Yale business school graduate and highly successful Silicon Valley entrepreneur and venture capitalist, who started Privateer Holdings in 2011 to focus on investment opportunities in the emerging legal marijuana business. He's since gone on to become one of the industry's recognized players, with millions in backing from Founders Fund, a $2 billion venture capital firm run by Peter Thiel, co-founder and former CEO of PayPal. At the time of the interview, though, Kennedy was still pretty green to the weed business.

"This is a more complicated industry than anything I've ever looked at by orders of magnitude," Kennedy informed me at the outset. "I've never worked this hard in my life, and I've never had this much fun."

To get up to speed before entering the field, Kennedy began his new venture with some "old-fashioned, boots-on-the-ground research," meeting with growers, lawyers, activists, dispensary owners, and other thought leaders of the trade, to pick their brains while looking for "smart people" to work with down the road. He found most companies to be "immature and unsophisticated," all of them competing in a fragmented market with terrible branding. "There were no institutional players. No Wall Street, no banks, no private equity, no venture capital.

And yet annual revenues were still $18 to $40 billion, with rapid growth."

Kennedy's point was that while the cannabis industry thrives wherever the law allows a free market in marijuana, things won't be truly *optimized* until a bunch of Yale business school types come in and take things over with their venture capital, private equity, and Wall Street leverage. So right off the bat it's important to note that the distinction being made is not between success and failure, but between making money and *making the most money possible no matter what.*

To be clear, I don't know anything about Brendan Kennedy personally, professionally, politically, or otherwise. He could conceivably be the most altruistic human being on Earth. And I've previously praised Privateer's first acquisition, a "Yelp-like" marijuana app called Leafly, as a vital resource for those interested in what the wisdom of the crowd has to say about specific strains of cannabis, or who want to make sure that the best-run marijuana stores and dispensaries are duly rewarded in the marketplace. But I'm decidedly less enthusiastic about the firm's next major play in the pot biz.

"We'd been approached by one million people about selling Bob Marley pipes, lighters, you name it," Rohan Marley told the *New Yorker*'s Andrew Marantz in 2014 for a story about Marley Natural, touted as the world's first global cannabis brand. "When I met this guy, I knew: This is the man."

What exactly drew the Marley family, and specifically serial entrepreneur (coffee, headphones, speakers, apparel) Rohan to Brendan Kennedy remains unclear, but it's not hard to understand the attraction going the other way. After all, there's a reason 1 million people have approached the scions of Bob seeking lucrative licensing deals. And it has a lot less to do with marijuana than with that other highly sought-after green.

"If you were to look for the most famous human being who

ever walked the face of the Earth related to cannabis," Kennedy boasted when announcing the licensing deal he brokered between Big Marley and Privateer, "it would be Bob Marley."

The Yale MBA went on to praise the dearly departed reggae superstar as a visionary. But a few years earlier, when Privateer acquired Leafly, Kennedy sang a far different tune.

"A big part of [Leafly's] appeal was that it wasn't already branded with symbols of pot culture," Kennedy explained in a *New York Times* story tellingly titled "How to Invest in Dope." "It didn't have any of the old clichés. The website wasn't plastered with pot leaves or pictures of Bob Marley."

Now, as you can probably tell from the number of times I've quoted or referenced Bob Marley already, he's someone I hold in the highest esteem as not just an artist but also as a razor-sharp critic of oppression, exploitation, and colonialism in all forms—military, political, cultural, financial, and otherwise. He also recognized the government, religion, and academia as just another mask for the establishment, and knew how to make that point in a way that's both visceral and easy to understand—as in his song "Babylon System."

Building church and university, deceiving the people continually

Me say them graduatin' thieves and murderers

Damn right. Because when you consider the real impact Wall Street has on the world, "Graduatin' Thieves and Murderers" might as well be written in Latin beneath the Yale business school crest. At least, that's how I tend to see things. Not that Rohan Marley needs to agree with me. But I do think that his father would plant his seeds elsewhere were he still alive to tend to the family's interests. Specifically, I'm guessing he'd rather support the longtime ganja growers among Jamaica's native Rastafarian community than fall in line with Privateer Holdings.

In fact, I'd like to believe Bob Marley would have been a guest of honor in rugged, mountainous West Jamaica the night respected Rasta elder Ras Iyah V called to order the first meeting of the Westmoreland Hemp and Ganja Farmers' Association—founded in 2014 to ensure that those who fought and struggled for decades for the legalization of cannabis don't get pushed aside when the Caribbean nation long known for producing high-quality herb inevitably begins to officially license growers and retailers.

"We will not stand by and watch people outside of Rastafari faith and grass-roots people take over this product," Iyah V declared in his opening remarks, to a loose semicircle of twenty-five hardscrabble Rastas, most of whom very seldom leave their clandestine ganja gardens out in the bush. "We are saying this loud and clear to the government, we are saying it to society, and we are saying it to the international community. Because we are not going to take baton licks and brutality and all of a sudden now when the legalization aspect come, let some rich people take it over—people who used to scoff and scorn at the very mention of the herb."

Iyah V has been working to help organize his fellow outlaw Rastafarian herbsmen into a legally recognized cannabis cooperative—one capable of proactively protecting their integrity and common interests amid the influx of big money expected to arrive along with legalization. In particular, Iyah V warns his brethren about the also newly formed Ganja Future Growers and Producers Association, which is backed by politically connected local business leaders, and wants to swoop in and take over Jamaica's marijuana industry just as soon as it becomes legal—a dynamic destined to play itself out whenever and wherever growing and selling marijuana moves into the mainstream economy.

Because at the risk of romanticizing the black market (never forget the cartels at the top of the pyramid!), just imagine the faith and dedication it takes for true believers in marijuana consciousness all over the world to not only grow and supply the herb under a brutal prohibition, but to then stick with it and try to come aboveground after a lifetime of paranoia and persecution—only to see the whole thing handed over to Babylon System, simply because capitalism tends to favor those with a lot of capital. That's certainly what happened to many of the mom-and-pop operations that thrived in the first wave of Colorado's "green rush," but then got edged out down the road by better-funded competitors who pushed for a set of regulations specifically designed to favor enterprises with plenty of cash on hand over those with deep roots and battle scars.

In "Get Rich or High Trying," I talked with business owners on both sides of that divide. Then I contacted Kris Krane, whom I first met more than ten years ago, when he worked at the National Organization for the Reform of Marijuana Laws (NORML). Later, as executive director of Students for Sensible Drug Policy, Kris helped inspire countless young people to begin fighting back against a War on Drugs that targets them so disproportionately. Before ultimately leaving full-time activism to enter the "private sector" as managing partner at 4Front Advisors, an Arizona-based consulting and investment firm focused on helping marijuana businesses nationwide open in full compliance with state and local law, while serving as a positive model for the industry.

Kris told me that while he surely misses the perhaps purer world of the nonprofit drug-law reform movement, he also sees his current work as an extension of those efforts. Because it's vitally important not just *that* we legalize marijuana in America and around the world, but also *how* we do so. Simply put, it's not nearly good enough for the new face of Big Marijuana to be a lot kinder and gentler than the Sinaloa Cartel. Not when we have a wholly unique opportunity to nurture a massive new American industry from the green shoots up. One that can break the Wall Street greed mold by embracing the higher ideals so many of us associate with getting high, like cooperation, compassion, creativity, empathy, innovation, inclusion, tolerance, and a feeling of interconnectedness that transcends the bottom line.

"Capitalism is definitely going to change cannabis, because until now it's been completely in the shadows and totally unregulated," Kris conceded, before offering a ray of hope. "At the same time, while I'm not idealistic enough to believe that legal cannabis will change the way that capitalism works and people behave, I do hope that within the cannabis industry, the way that things are rolling out will provide us with a buffer period to get it right. Obviously, if cannabis were made completely legal at the federal level and in every state all at once, the big alcohol and tobacco companies would swoop in and dominate the market by resorting to the same tactics they use in their core businesses, but that's not what's happening. Instead we're seeing cannabis legalized state-by-state, thus keeping those kinds of players largely on the sidelines."

Which says to me that if we want to see a cannabis industry that's as progressive, innovative, compassionate, and downright revolutionary as the marijuana culture it serves, it's up to those of us with a stakeholder's interest to get directly involved—right quick. And that's especially true for all the young people on Earth who see getting high as a natural extension of *their* highest ideals.

Besides, what could be more fun and rewarding than selling weed—without selling out?

HOW TO START YOUR CANNABIS CAREER

From entry level to executive level, wholly unique opportunities now exist to get in early on the next great global industry. And that includes not just tens of thousands of "green jobs" directly related to the cultivation, processing, and distribution of marijuana but also all the ancillary businesses involved, including real estate, construction, security, research, marketing, design, travel, hospitality, events, media, technology, and more.

"The Silicon Valley of cannabis is already happening," Troy Dayton, cofounder of the ArcView Group, once told me during a meeting of the angel investor network, which functions like a *Shark Tank* for weed. "The hippies were right about personal computing, alternative energy, organic foods, and yoga—four of the biggest business success stories of the past few decades—and they're right again about cannabis. All of this bubbles up from the counterculture, until finally the mainstream takes notice."

And yet a crazy kind of catch-22 exists whereby if you haven't worked in the pot business until now, you've got no experience and no track record, and if you have previously worked in the pot business, you probably broke the law to do so—either of which can make it tough to get a foot in the door, especially since, just as in the black market, most employers in the aboveground weed industry still prefer to hire someone they know, or, failing that, someone who's at least vouched for by someone they know. So assuming *you* don't know anyone in the marijuana game, how do you get some playing time and prove yourself?

"Most cannabusinesses don't advertise job openings, so a proactive approach will yield the best results," Steve DeAngelo, Dayton's partner in cofounding the ArcView Group, advises. "Compile a list of the local places you'd like to work and then call them and let them know you'd like to drop off a cover letter and résumé. Be polite and professional at all times, but don't be afraid to be persistent as well."

DeAngelo, who also operates America's largest medical-marijuana dispensary—Harborside Health Center in Oakland, California—says he asks each prospective employee the same question: *What role has cannabis played in your life?*

"I'm hoping to hear something like: 'I absolutely love cannabis—it's taught me many lessons and helped me develop as a person. Nothing would make me happier than working all day with this plant.' So always remember to emphasize your devotion to cannabis and willingness to work hard and learn, no matter how much you already know. And always describe your previous experience using objective and professional language, with a focus on specific skills you've developed. For example, instead of saying, 'I dealt massive weed to pay my way through college,' you might try: 'I developed extensive product knowledge and negotiating techniques during ten years as an independent cannabis broker. During that time I initiated supplier and customer relationships, while managing all quality control, security, and accounting.'"

Start your marijuana job search like any other quest for employment, by making a realistic assessment of your skills, knowledge, and experience. Then zero in on positions that match. But first, divorce yourself from any notion that because the marijuana industry has been marginalized for so long, it will be an easier hill to climb than getting ahead in some other, more straitlaced, field. The fact is that all the extra baggage and bullshit that goes along with selling a barely legal herb actually makes it that much harder to get ahead. And despite all the rapid growth in the industry, the pot job market is now and will always be tight, precisely because it's so much more fun, rewarding, and worthwhile to be part of Big Marijuana than to make sprockets and cogs for the man.

So here's a few job-hunting tips to get you started:

- A prospective employer in the marijuana industry wants to like you, but *needs* to trust you, so work hard to prove yourself as a knowledgeable, capable, diligent professional first and a fun person to get blazed with second.

- Dress codes and office culture can vary widely in the marijuana industry, usually landing somewhere between "casual Friday all week" and "no shoes, no shirt, no problem." So find a place that matches your own sense of style, and you'll have one less thing to worry about.

- Don't show up for a job interview (or for work) high and/or smelling of cannabis (unless your boss does too).

- Don't ever blame a personal shortcoming on cannabis use. For instance, if there's a typo on your résumé, and you respond with, "Oh man, I must have been really stoned when I did that," you are (a) making excuses rather than taking responsibility (b) disrespecting yourself (c) disrespecting the herb, and (d) not getting the job.

- Never confuse passion for knowledge when it comes to the cannabis plant. Meaning that how much you love to get high, how often you get high, and how high you get are all fairly irrelevant data points to an employer compared to how much you know about cannabis, and how hard you're willing to work at learning even more.

* Consider attending a quality marijuana trade school near where you live to gain valuable skills and business contacts, but also look out for shady, fly-by-night operations that charge large fees for "insider" knowledge that's either wrong, easily obtained from the Internet for free, or both. Start your assessment by taking a critical look at who's running the school and what else they've done in the industry.

* Becoming actively engaged in the marijuana movement is another great way to establish yourself as someone with passion and persistence when it comes to working with the plant, while making important local connections. "If you've been an activist in the cannabis law-reform movement, that's always a big plus," according to DeAngelo. "It demonstrates character and commitment."

* If you live in a place without taxed, regulated marijuana cultivation and retail sales, plan a fact-finding visit to a state where you can legally tour cannabis cultivation facilities, stores, and other ancillary businesses. Send emails and make phone calls in advance of your trip in order to meet with as many people as possible while in town.

* Cannabusiness culture remains a bit laid-back, and we aim to keep it that way, so when meeting people casu-

ally (that is, not at a formal job interview) don't "network," just make friends. Remember, marijuana offers those with the right mind-set a unique ability to see through the bullshit in life, so if your only motivation is "what's in it for me?" and it comes with a side of pushy, overaggressive self-promotion, that's likely to prove counterproductive.

⚕ Always have a lighter handy. Always have rolling papers handy. You just never know!

NOW *HIGH*-ERING: TEN LEGAL POT JOBS

From budtenders, cultivators, and trimmers to inventory specialists, product buyers, and marketing managers, marijuana businesses large and small employ people at all levels, and always look to hire those with a real passion for the plant.

Budtender

Typically an entry-level position, budtenders work behind the counter at a retail cannabis store or a medical-marijuana dispensary, interacting with customers, offering point-of-purchase information, and processing orders. Ideally, budtenders have a wealth of knowledge about cannabis and its effects so they can offer clear, fact-based advice to customers who may be largely or wholly unfamiliar with the varying effects of different strains, *indica*s and *sativa*s, and alternate means of ingestion like vapor, tincture, edibles, and dabbing.

Budtenders should be patient, enjoy working with the public, and love teaching people about cannabis. Many stores and dispensaries promote from within, so the best budtenders tend to move up in the organization after first learning the ropes from the very center of the action.

Cultivator

I know, I know, you've been growing *the best* marijuana on Earth in your basement for years, and now you're ready to show the world who's the real King of Cannabis. And how do I know that? Because during my ten years working at *High Times* I must have met a thousand different pot growers, and they all fell into one of two camps—total newbies, and those who grow *the best* weed in the world.

But does that mean you're ready to move from four lights in the basement to designing, constructing, and overseeing a 25,000-square-foot facility in a converted warehouse space? Let's be honest, probably not. So you better sit down, because I've got some rough news.

Turns out, one of the very few drawbacks of marijuana legalization is the unavoidable fact that, as prohibition falls, the world will continue to smoke roughly the same amount of herb—and maybe even more—but far fewer people will make a living growing all those lovely buds, mostly because of automation and economies of scale. Sure, the lucky and talented few who end up running large-scale, legal, licensed commercial operations will make bank in this new paradigm, but at the same time every giant bud factory puts a hundred little guys out of business. We may even reach the point where Willie Nelson has to perform a special Farm Aid concert to support his favorite kind of farmers.

Again, not to romanticize the black market and all its depredations, but how many other crops can you grow in a corner of your basement, without any type of license or accreditation, and still earn enough cash to pay off a modest mortgage while making steady deposits into the kids' college fund? Zero. But then again, those high black-market prices only exist because of what's called the prohibition tax, which underground growers, smugglers, and dealers add to the cost of illicit herb as payment for the serious risks they take.

"Growers who are against legalization are harvesting bad karma," medical-marijuana activist and cannabis entrepreneur Richard Lee told me flatly in 2010, when I interviewed him during his ultimately failed campaign to legalize marijuana in California via ballot initiative Prop 19. "When somebody else gets busted, that's the subsidy that keeps prices high—that, and the violence down in Mexico."

All of which means, and here comes the rough news, that if you want to come in from the cold and start growing weed legally, you're going to have to accept that the high margins of the black market won't be following you. Make no mistake, there's plenty of profit to be made if you really are the best of the best, but if not, just stop and consider the vast difference in salary between, for example, the nation's leading vintners, and the folks in the field who actually water and pick the grapes.

The good news is that if you've got a green thumb, a detail-oriented mind-set, and solid experience cultivating this plant, you can find a place to legally make money by helping marijuana grow and flourish. Imagine waking up every morning and knowing that the day's major responsibilities include watering, fertilizing, inspecting, and harvesting cannabis. Imagine sleeping peacefully at night, secure in the knowledge that the cops won't break down the door at dawn looking for your grow room. Doesn't that sound nice?

Trimmer

By the time they reach your grinder, top-grade marijuana buds look like miniature bonsai trees, but they don't start off that way. First the plants must be stripped of their large fan leaves, followed by a thorough, precise manicuring session to remove the smaller leaves and trim the buds themselves into perfect little nuggets. Done to the highest standards, it's a painstaking, time-consuming job.

Most large-scale legal marijuana growers now harvest and trim year-round, which means there's steady work if you're good with scissors, have excellent focus, and don't mind sitting in one place all day. You won't learn the business the same way you might as a budtender, but it's a great foot in the door if you're interested in cultivation, while earning a solid hourly wage without having to deal with anybody at work except Ms. Mary Jane herself.

Edibles

Marijuana-infused food, or edibles, is the fastest-growing segment of the cannabis industry right now, and there's still plenty of room to get involved at every level. So anyone with a strong culinary background, or extensive experience in commercial food preparation and distribution, should consider edibles as a way to get a foothold in the marijuana business. There's also a pressing need for those capable of overseeing production, inventory, marketing, packaging, branding, social media outreach, promotions, and all other necessary aspects of running a packaged-goods business (that just happens to sell intoxicating peanut brittle).

Start by learning everything you can about the science of making and ingesting edibles, from how to create various cannabis infusions of a uniform potency to proper dosage, safe usage, and what to do in the event of an overdose. Try as many edibles currently on the market as possible (just not all at once!), and take careful notes about what you like and don't like about each. Research the market as well, studying up on production methods, pricing, distribution, and anywhere you see an underserved customer base. Then identify the existing edibles companies you'd most like to work for, or make a plan for creating your own.

Topicals

Most marijuana topicals don't get you high, though a few companies make massage oils and "feminine enhancement products" in concentrations potent enough to confer a mild buzz through transdermal absorption. For the most part, however, the healing power of cannabis topicals remains within the skin and the underlying muscles. Still, there's huge upside potential for this market.

From entry-level positions mixing up batches of marijuana-infused hand cream and lip balm to ditching the corporate world for a chance at building the Body Shop of cannabis skin-care products from the ground up, pot legalization has opened up a wide variety of opportunities. Best of all, this often-overlooked niche has emerged as a rare female-centric sector of the all-too-male-dominated marijuana business. So if you're turned off by some of the macho bro culture around growing and selling weed, or you're looking for a less well-established part of the industry with plenty of room to grow as marijuana becomes increasingly legal and accepted, definitely investigate topicals— ideally starting with a canna-spa day spent pampering yourself with the highest quality lotions, oils, balms, creams, and ointments you can find!

Concentrate Artist

As noted previously, the "most explosive" trend in cannabis to-day is extremely concentrated cannabis extracts called dabs, which are made by using a chemical solvent to strip marijuana's cannabinoids and terpinoids away from the surrounding plant matter so they can be ingested in a highly purified form. This technique has been around for decades, but became popular only in the last five years, so there's a huge demand for skilled professionals who know how to perform these chemical extractions safely and effectively. Several states already allow those with proper know-how and equipment to become licensed makers of concentrates, and hopefully that trend will continue, as it's the only way to take this process out of the shadows and put it into the hands of those who know what they're doing.

So if you love cannabis and have an advanced degree in lab science, you might consider looking into how these extractions work by touring a licensed facility in a legal state. And if you're a backyard black-market concentrate artist getting by on the fringes, stop now, and go get a degree in organic chemistry so you can start making dabs safely and legally.

🌿 PRO TIP 🌿

FOLLOW YOUR BLISS

"Selling pot allowed me to get through college and make enough money to start off in comedy."

—BILL MAHER, *BUSINESSWEEK*

Cannabis Buyer

What's more fun than treating yourself to a nice fat sack of weed come payday? How about buying hundreds of pounds of weed every week, from some of the best cultivators in your area, with someone else's money? Because that's the basic job description for a cannabis buyer at a medical-marijuana dispensary or retail pot store.

First you schedule meetings with various top-level growers who'd like to sell you their finest herb at a fair wholesale price, then each of them shows up at an appointed hour bearing a sample of their merchandise for inspection—including tests for potency, contaminants, aroma, visual appeal, taste, and overall wonderfulness. Until finally, if everything's up to snuff, a price is negotiated, payment is made, and the goods change hands with hearty congratulations all around, and perhaps a celebratory toke to seal the deal.

Like I said, nice work if you can get it. The hardest part of the gig, of course, is telling a rightfully proud grower that you're just not able to make an offer on their herb. Sometimes the quality isn't up to standards, but often it's because you've got a glut of that particular strain already, or you're overstocked in general and only looking for something you can sell at a higher or lower price point to balance the menu. So there's a lot more to the job than just knowing what makes for top-quality herb— you also need to understand how to manage the shop's inventory effectively, respond to feedback from customers, and keep a bunch of unruly growers in line.

Which means being a buyer is definitely not a job for the faint of heart, and not one that's easily obtained either. Unless you've already got a name in the weed business (legal or otherwise), this is a position you should aspire to, not apply for. But *man oh man*, it's nice to dream.

Dispensary Management

Whether you own a dispensary or operate one on behalf of someone else, there's no place the rubber meets the road in the world of legal marijuana more directly than when you're running a storefront retail outlet. You've got to deal with growers, wholesalers, customers, employees, investors, government regulators, and your industry peers on a daily basis—all while operating under a powerful microscope of public scrutiny. Plus, there's the heavy burden of knowing that any screw-ups you make could potentially affect not just your own business and the lives of your clients and colleagues but also the entire marijuana movement. Because those who inexplicably find cannabis abhorrent to the point of banning it are just waiting to seize on the smallest fuck-up to make another run at our rights and freedoms.

That said, this industry does desperately need more dedicated, energetic small business owners interested in putting the cannabis community first. Too many retail outlets do a fine job of keeping the shelves stocked and the cash registers ringing but only make a passing effort at educating and politically organizing their customers, which marks a huge missed opportunity on both the micro and the macro level. So if you want to sell pot *properly*, don't delay, opportunity is knocking right now.

Tourism and Events

Already, a small number of tour groups, cannabis-friendly hotels, and marijuana-centric events have sprouted up in legalization states to service those eager to take a "jay-cation" in the land of the free. And as this particular strain of green tourism continues to grow and evolve, a plethora of job opportunities will open up along with it.

Think about it this way: Wine tourism in California's Napa Valley currently generates more than $1 billion in spending every year, even though alcohol is perfectly legal and widely available everywhere in the country. Now imagine living in Oklahoma, loving cannabis, and facing harsh punishment every day for simply having a joint in your pocket or a roach in your ashtray at home. Wouldn't you want to board an airplane for a short, domestic flight to a magical realm where you're instantly transformed from a hardened, dangerous criminal into a coveted tourist ready to pump a little money into the local economy?

And I see cannabis tourism as not just a huge growth industry but also a fine way to spread a positive marijuana message around the world when all those lucky tourists go home and brag to their friends. So if you're a people person *and* a pot person, what could be better than making sure someone's dream weed vacation exceeds all expectations?

Media

For about a hundred years, the media has basically shit the bed royally when it comes to marijuana. Yes, the government lied, and continues to lie, but that's what governments do, and everybody knows it. Which is why, in theory, we rely on a free and independent press to publish the truth and safeguard our liberties, no matter who it offends.

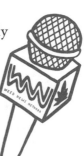

Anyone looking for a textbook case of how the modern media catastrophically fails in that watchdog role, however, need look no further than the atrocious reporting on marijuana that began back in the days of William Randolph Hearst and continues today (though things *have* markedly improved ever since the "right people" started making money off this herb). The good news is that the corporate media's complete failure to understand cannabis culture actually represents a tremendous opportunity for grass-roots-level, marijuana-centric media to step up and inform the world about this most miraculous herb. So if you're into writing, photography, videography, social media, or some new form of mass communication that old codgers like me haven't even heard about yet, start your own marijuana media empire today by getting online and putting your best information out there where people can access it. Don't worry about making money at first—just learn the skills you need, attract an audience, and burnish your reputation as a provider of engaging, real stories about this plant and those who love it. In time, you'll either find a way to transform that passion into revenue, or you'll land a job with a media company that values your well-honed talents and unique point of view.

BUY LOW, SELL HIGH: THE PERILOUS WORLD OF POT STOCKS

In August 2013, the Financial Industry Regulatory Authority issued an official alert regarding the high potential for fraud among marijuana stocks:

> *The con artists behind marijuana stock scams may try to entice investors with optimistic and potentially false and misleading information that in turn creates unwarranted demand for shares*

of small, thinly traded companies that often have little or no history of financial success. The scammers behind these "pump and dump" scams can then sell off their shares, leaving investors with worthless stock.

Then in an April 2014 article titled "Inside the Pot Stock Bubble," *Forbes* staff writer Nathan Vardi profiled "the shady band of ex-cons, ganja-preneurs and multilevel marketers behind the great pot penny-stock boom," reporting,

With Colorado and Washington now permitting the sale of marijuana for recreational use, and 20 states allowing it medically, some 60 publicly traded outfits, many snarled in a tangled, difficult-to-track web of interconnections, have popped up, claiming to be pot and hemp stocks. Almost none, mind you, emerged via an IPO and all the pesky disclosure and scrutiny that come with that path. Instead, real estate, marketing and oil outfits have miraculously morphed into medical marijuana and hemp companies, either through reverse mergers or simply changing their declared line of business. And just about every single one is thinly traded on the over-the-counter bulletin board, or Pink Sheets, where promoters can push them with the enthusiasm of a campus dealer.

So while there's certainly potentially lucrative investment opportunities out there in marijuana, don't ever let your faith in the beneficent power of pot blind you when it comes to handing over your money. Not when you're buying a bag of weed in the parking lot outside a Tom Petty concert, and definitely not when making a major (or even minor) financial investment. And even if a company's financials do add up, and based on a full and transparent analysis of their prospects you reasonably expect a significant return on your investment, you've still got to ask yourself if the enterprise you're planning to back really deserves the money. In short, does the investment benefit the cannabis community, or just your pocketbook? Because smoking pot properly absolutely precludes making a fast buck off the backs of your fellow herbalists.

MARIJUANA SHOULD TRANSFORM CAPITALISM, NOT THE OTHER WAY AROUND

While every other segment of the economy is already tightly controlled by Big Money and deeply entrenched interests, marijuana remains, for the moment, wide open. Which means cannabis legalization offers a wholly unique opportunity to reshape the global economy by building a truly progressive industry from the ground up—one that addresses income inequality, workers' rights, the environment, and unchecked corporate power.

So here's a few simple suggestions for making sure the weed heads prevail over the greed heads:

* Since both marijuana's biggest supporters and biggest detractors fear the rise of Big Marijuana, we must build this odd-bedfellows coalition into an effective means of making sure all regulation of the cannabis industry specifically supports small, local, socially responsible businesses over large, corporate, mercenary interests.

* No nonviolent marijuana offender, felon or otherwise, should ever be barred from participation in the legal

marijuana business. Such bans are not only an additional slap in the face to those who've already suffered needless punishment, they also push some of the most knowledgeable and ethical growers and cannabusinesspeople back into the shadows.

- Every person working in the cannabis industry should make a living wage, guaranteed by a minimum wage for the industry that's significantly higher than what the state requires.

- All cannabis retailers, recreational or medicinal, should be required to supply a significant portion of their inventory for free to low-income people in the community with serious ailments and no means to pay for the cannabis they need. For example, in Berkeley, California, medical-marijuana dispensaries must provide 2 percent of their cannabis at no charge to individual patients who make under $32,000, or families that earn less than $46,000, and that free herb must be "the same quality on average as medical cannabis that is dispensed to other members."

- No tax should be imposed on marijuana that's not imposed on alcohol. And no tax monies collected for marijuana growing, distribution, and sales should be used to fund law enforcement, anti-marijuana public-relations campaigns, or the private addiction treatment industry (which for decades has preyed on marijuana users forced into rehab by the criminal-justice system). Instead, invest in programs like public education, or better yet, serious scientific research into the medicinal efficacy of cannabis.

⚹ Marijuana advertising and promotion should be held to a high standard and serve an educational function, rather than following the alcohol model of using scantily clad women to promote overconsumption.

⚹ Those profiting off this herb in one state must financially support the fight to legalize it in other states—if not in acknowledgment of their obvious responsibility to support our shared fight for freedom, then at least in their own narrow self-interest as a business that must truly keep expanding or else risk a dangerous backlash.

LEGAL WEED IS ONLY THE BEGINNING

When I first became involved in cannabis activism twenty years ago, people invariably asked: *Why waste your time trying to legalize marijuana? It's never going to happen.* Well, it's happening now, and the story of how an underfunded, widely mocked, willfully disregarded movement came out on top should serve to inform and inspire any effort to take on the system and win. So what lessons can other progressive political movements learn from pot?

⚹ First you shift public opinion, then you change the law or reform the system, because without broad-based political support it's impossible to make serious political change. Thirty years ago, marijuana legalization made just as much sense as it does now, but at that

time immediate legislative progress was not possible—
only public outreach and education.

⚕ Have patience, faith, and perseverance when going up
against the government, Big Business, and entrenched
interests. The public responds not just to facts and effective messaging but to consistency as well, which
means it may take a long time of using the same tactics
before your message starts to break through.

⚕ Don't change your position to reach a consensus, just
stay firm and bring the consensus to you through
clear, consistent framing of the issue. For example, by
focusing on the fact that marijuana is less harmful than
alcohol, and therefore should be treated the same, reformers in Colorado taught the public to view cannabis in a new way, and then form their own opinions.

⚕ Nurture the grassroots, so they can spread your message. That's how the marijuana movement has managed to prevail in America without the support of
either major political party. Remember, most people
will listen to a politician, but they will *believe* a friend,
relative, or coworker, provided that you have a real
command of the facts and convey them effectively.

⚕ Activism works best when it's fun, otherwise people
burn out or wander off. So the marijuana movement
learned to use every political activity as a chance to
socialize, and also to make sure every massive smoke-
out had a political element.

THE BOTTOM LINE

When it comes to how to get ahead in cannabusiness, never, ever forget these invaluable words of wisdom from the immortal Fabulous Furry Freak Brothers:

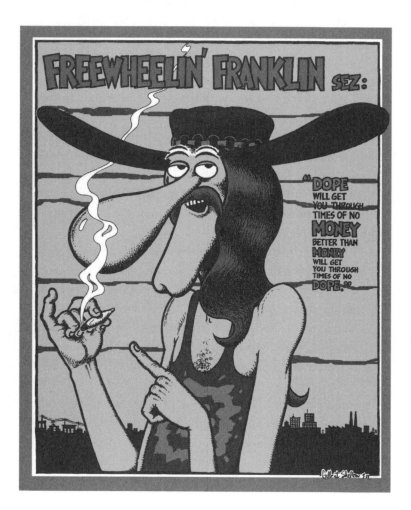

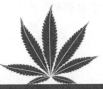

CHAPTER 6

The High Road: Travel

*There's no better way to see the world
than through a pair of red eyes.*

A while back, I spent about four months down in Costa Rica while working on a book. Mostly I stayed at an amazing off-the-grid permaculture farm on a largely uninhabited stretch of the Caribbean coast, but I also took some time to scout around and see the country, plus one really disastrous trip to Panama involving bad shellfish.

I'd never traveled alone and without an itinerary before, and quickly learned that such wandering requires making a journey not just into the world, but also into the self.

For despite the obvious romantic appeal of taking a "radical sabbatical" in paradise, I actually found myself at a rather daunting personal crossroads at that time, with the path ahead still unclear. And so, upon arrival in the fun-loving, herb-friendly little surf town of Puerto Viejo, I kept largely to the edges and outskirts—more than happy to swim, eat, drink, think, smoke weed, read a book, and otherwise enjoy the solitary pleasures of a loner stoner while largely going unnoticed.

Until one day, just before sunset, I followed a narrow foot-path through the jungle and down to the beach. I lit a fat joint, planning to smoke half immediately, and save the rest for later, when a strange figure approached in the twilight. Bald, short, scrawny, skin weathered to the look of old leather, with a small pack of mangy dogs at his feet, the man approached cautiously and asked about the paperback novel I was holding. Then, after a few hits off my spliff, he grew quite animated, and volunteered that he used to be a pot smuggler back in the 1970s, as a way to fund his frequent surfing trips to exotic locales. Surfing and smuggling, my new friend Patrick explained, went hand in hand in those days.

"Certainly it's a symbiotic relationship," he told me. "Surfers can't work because we have to go surfing, but we still need to earn a living. It was also my cover story—whenever anybody asked what I was doing in Africa, Colombia, the Cayman Islands, or wherever, I just said 'surfing.' It was like getting paid to go on vacation, basically. And meanwhile, marijuana teaches you to be in the moment. You almost become molecular when you smoke good ganja—an invisible part of your surroundings—and that's a key skill for a smuggler to master."

I didn't out myself as a journalist that night, never mind a marijuana journalist, but old habits do die hard, and so I ended up pretty much interviewing him on the spot, at first to see if I could poke any holes in his tall tale, and then out of sheer fascination. As we finished the joint, and moved on to taking slugs off a small bottle of rum he fished out of a worn tote bag, Patrick told me he was raised as a ward of the state of New York because his mother conceived him illegitimately while her husband was fighting in Europe during World War II. Fourteen years later, mother and child were finally reunited, only to be torn apart again by a draft notice for Vietnam, where the small, scrappy, perpetually stoned nineteen-year-old soldier dodged bullets and took shrapnel, returning home in one piece, with a satchel of smuggled marijuana as a souvenir.

"You see, I was a radioman, and the Ziploc bag that we now take for granted had just been invented to keep things dry in the jungles of Vietnam," he explained, relating the origin of his first black-market venture, which involved buying ganja from Vietnamese growers and selling it to his fellow soldiers. "The batteries for my radio were very sensitive, so I always had a few extra Ziploc bags. That made me very popular."

After an honorable discharge, Patrick set out in search of his own *Endless Summer*, with a small-time smuggling business on the side that initially was meant to merely subsidize his far-flung surfing trips but soon flowered into a high-flying international enterprise all its own—at least, until an unlucky break left him washed up for two years in a Caribbean prison.

Upon release, the ex-con, who took to calling himself Captain Zero, decided to leave the underworld behind and simply vanish—at first sending a series of cryptic postcards to friends and family back in the States, then drifting away completely, like a huge wave pulled back by the undertow. Several years passed without any word before an old smuggling associate turned author named Allan Weisbecker finally set out to find him, a journey later chronicled in the surf-lit classic *In Search of Captain Zero*.

"I've become kind of like mythology since Allen's book came out," Patrick told me, with obvious relish. "If I was having an identity crisis before, at least I have another identity to fall back on now. I have people from eighteen to eighty, from Oklahoma to Berlin, come and find me, and I'm humbled by it. I meet people from all over the world, with different philosophies, ideologies, religions, occupations, and everything else. I call them my living libraries."

Classifying himself as a leisure consultant, Patrick says he now gets by teaching tightly wound tourists how to relax and "surf by their senses," which on any given day could involve "lounging on the beach, collecting shells, hiking to breathtaking vistas, snorkeling, drinking and laughing with locals at tucked-away cantinas, biking down country roads, chasing monkeys, and Lord only knows what else." He chooses his clients carefully by first observing them from afar, then engaging them in friendly conversation, before ever offering his services. As I wrote in a *High Times* cover story:

> Captain Zero wants to be your leisure consultant. But first, you have to make your own way down to Puerto Viejo, Costa Rica, because this travel package includes neither flight, nor accommodations. Once you arrive, however, the Captain will be more than happy to help you find a nice place to stay, in any price range, not to mention a secluded beach, gnarly waves, hiking trails deep into the jungle, the best cheap eats, and an out of the way, seaside cantina where you can sip a rum and puff a fat joint, while a reggae band plays to a packed house of irie locals.
>
> By the way, no need for advance reservations. You can locate the Captain almost any time of day or night in this small surfer hideaway, whether he's taking his coffee and scouting out the breaks first thing in the morning from the shade of the lifeguard stand, coasting through the two-street town on his iconic yellow bicycle (conveniently outfitted with a machete holder), or leading his entourage of semi-stray dogs through the narrow footpaths along the shoreline by the light of his trusty flashlight. Track him down all on your own, or ask just about anyone you meet along the way for help.

If you do make contact with this legendary herbsman, please say hi (*high*) for me, and then by all means sign up as a leisure consulting client, and let the captain take you along for a private tour of paradise with the ultimate freewheeling guide. Forget about set itineraries, tourist traps, and overpriced "excursions," and get ready for life lived in the moment, navigating the swells of existence with a man who's turned the eternal balancing act of the wave rider into his own higher calling.

During my time under his tutelage, Captain Zero didn't just introduce me to the little town he's called home for more than twenty years—since long before electricity arrived, and back when making a phone call involved a full day of travel. He also taught me a new way to see the world, both while out wandering and even back at home. Because making a journey into the self doesn't have to start by crawling straight up your own ass or hiding behind a book all the time. Unless, you know, it's *this* book—then by all means, carry on.

THE HIGH-MINDED WANDERER

Follow the rules of the high road when it comes to finding, acquiring, transporting, and enjoying cannabis safely when away from home.

- Always know the law where you are now and where you're going next. Making an informed decision to risk a fine, arrest, or worse for cannabis is one thing, but don't ever blindly blunder your way into big trouble.

- Respect local customs at all times. For instance, in Amsterdam, it's perfectly lovely to light up in a coffeeshop, but not so in the street. In India, some areas strictly prohibit cannabis, and others allow licensed *bhang* shops to operate openly.

⚕ When buying marijuana in places where it's legal, don't settle for the first store you see or the closest one to where you're staying. Instead, seek out a retailer with a solid reputation for both high-quality cannabis and enthusiastic customer service.

⚕ If you're involved in cannabis activism where you live (and you should be!), make contact with fellow activists where you're traveling and ask for recommendations. Odds are they'll probably offer to show you around a bit. I've met some really cool friends and had some amazing fun this way!

⚕ When traveling for business, never assume that your coworkers, clients, employees, contractors, and so on are cool with weed, or even cool with being asked if they're cool with weed. And this remains true even when visiting states that have legalized it. Just as at a company-wide team-building meeting in Nevada, you probably shouldn't mention your plan to visit a brothel later that night.

FLYING HIGH

In 2011, Indiana rapper Freddie Gibbs took to Twitter to recount an amusing run-in with the federal Transportation Security Administration (TSA), posting—"TSA found my weed, and let me keep it. They just left me a note. 'C'mon son.' LOL"—plus a photo of the note and the weed.

Your mileage may vary, however, as official TSA policy clearly stipulates that while "TSA security officers do not search for marijuana or other drugs, in the event a substance that appears to be marijuana is observed during security screening, TSA will refer the matter to a law enforcement officer." And that applies even if you're flying from one legal state to another, since TSA is governed by federal law.

The good news, though, is that if you can prove you're in compliance with state law (at least in the state you're standing in, if not your final destination), and you're only carrying a personal amount of cannabis, then local law enforcement likely won't give you a hard time. And TSA may just wave you on as well.

"They're not looking for small amounts of weed," quipped comedian Ngaio Bealum to the *San Francisco Chronicle*. "They're looking for 'a bomb' not 'the bomb.'"

Keep in mind, this all applies strictly to domestic flights, as anything international involves going through customs, and that's a whole other level of bureaucracy to deal with. So as always, the key is to know the law where you are, where you're going, and anywhere you're scheduled to stop in between. And if you do decide to bring some herb along for the ride, pack it in a vacuum sealer, wrap it in your medical-marijuana recommendation if you have one, and hide it somewhere clever in your luggage. I could make specific recommendations, but then what if this book fell into the wrong hands?

SHOULD I EAT A POT BROWNIE BEFORE BOARDING THE PLANE?

The short answer to this question is a resounding *no*, but only because you had to ask, if that makes sense.

Basically, hurtling through space, stuck in a metal tube, wedged between two total strangers like sardines in a can for hours on end while high as fuck on edibles is not for everybody. Just the fact that you're wondering if that's a good plan or not means it's definitely not a good one, because while the idea of vibing out on the flight, watching a dumb movie, having a few laughs, and then sleeping it off peacefully may sound highly appealing, the potential downside's just too steep for those who go too far and freak out at 30,000 feet. The best-case scenario in that instance is you manage to white-knuckle it the rest of the flight without unduly alarming anyone onboard with your wild eyes and erratic behavior. Worst case, you shit your pants and yammer gibberish until they divert the plane.

So, naturally, if you've been a "frequent flier" when it comes to edibles and air travel for many years, and never had a problem, then more power to you. But otherwise, as much as I love marijuana, I just wouldn't recommend it for anxiety relief or general enhancement in this instance. Still, if you do get high before the flight—even just a last joint before heading into the terminal—make sure to pack a delicious sandwich in your carry-on bag instead of relying on whatever they've got on the plane.

You'll thank me later!

STONELY PLANET: A LEGAL WEED TRAVEL GUIDE

As marijuana legalization spreads like a grassfire, so too does the rapidly growing cannabis tourism industry, which offers kindhearted travelers from around the world everything from 420-friendly airport transfers, privately catered cannabis-infused gourmet meals, and ganja-themed "Bud-and-Breakfasts" to guided excursions at leading marijuana retail shops, cultivation centers, and edibles-manufacturing facilities. There's also now a slew of special events every year geared to herbal enthusiasts, from cups, concerts, and festivals to business conferences and political rallies.

So if you're ready to experience legal weed for yourself—up close and personal—first spend some time deciding the right destination and when to go. Ideally, book a trip that you'd love to take anyway (skiing in Colorado, fly-fishing in Oregon), and then look for ways to immerse yourself in the local herb scene upon arrival. If you opt to make arrangements through a pot tourism company, definitely look into their offerings before signing up, as the quality of these tours (and the outfits providing them) varies widely. And if you decide to choose your own adventure instead, don't be shy about calling up some local cannabusinesses in advance to see if they'll make time to give you a tour.

In the meantime, I'm more than happy to share a few of my own fairly random, totally subjective travel tips for the world's best-loved *jay*-cation destinations, most of which I've been lucky enough to visit on multiple occasions.

Denver

Ever since Colorado became the first state to open legal recreational marijuana stores on January 1, 2014, the (sigh) Mile-High City of Denver has pretty much served as the capital of Marijuanaland. So there's lots to see and do, including visiting some of the world's largest and most sophisticated cannabusinesses. On the way into town from the airport, you can stop at **Medicine Man** and take a tour of their on-site 40,000-square-foot cultivation facility, followed by a trip to the showroom to purchase a sampling of cannabis, concentrates, and edibles. Just don't blow your whole bud budget at the very first stop!

As for accommodations, if you've got some money to burn (along with all that herb you just bought), book a room at the **Warwick Denver Hotel,** one of the few centrally located luxury hotels in the city with balconies (call ahead to confirm). Or better yet, investigate Denver's growing number of Bud-and-Breakfast options for a less pricey and far more personal experience that's also a great way to connect with pot-friendly locals and your fellow ganja tourists.

And once you've checked in and gotten stoned, what's next? Hopefully something amazing to eat!

The good news is that by all local accounts, the legalization of marijuana has had a hugely positive effect on the city's food scene. For breakfast, you've pretty much gotta hit **Snooze**—Denver's leading brunch spot—for a "pancake flight" of three different highly innovative takes on the flapjack. For a budget lunch with a 420-friendly vibe, try **Cheba Hut,** a marijuana-themed sandwich shop (yup, they're "toasted") that serves surprisingly good food, has a full bar, and cranks thirty-seven-minute Phish jams in the middle of the afternoon. And for dinner, head over to **Domo,** which consistently ranks among America's top-rated Asian restaurants by stuffing you full of "Japanese country food" at very reasonable prices. I also like Domo because there's a beautiful garden seating area in the back, and plenty of space in the roomy parking lot to have a discreet smoke before stepping inside.

As for music, nightlife, and adventure, start by consulting the Cannabist, a marijuana-centric website created and operated by the *Denver Post.* Each week, Susan Squibb, the Cannabist's resident advice columnist, posts a comprehensive list of pot-friendly goings-on around town. Personally, I usually end up making my way to **Quixote's True Blue**, a Grateful Dead–themed bar that wins my affection for its excellent live music bookings (usually on two stages at once), its highly accommodating outdoor area, and, of course, its Ping-Pong table. Also, don't ever miss a chance to see a concert at **Red Rocks,** a truly breathtaking outdoor amphitheater about thirty minutes outside Denver. And be sure to check out one of the herb-friendly stand-up comedy nights promoted by Kayvan Khalatbari, of Denver Relief, under his **Sex Pot** comedy umbrella.

Colorado Highlight: Telluride Mushroom Festival

Colorado has long been a huge tourist draw for skiers, mountain bikers, hikers, and other outdoor enthusiasts, and it's no secret that those who truly love nature often love a natural high as well. Personally, I don't ski, but a few years ago I made a pilgrimage to Telluride in August for the annual mushroom festival. The town itself combines the charm of the Old West with a modern take on good vibes, sustainable living, and amazing ganja, while the festival explores fungi in all aspects, including culinary, medicinal, industrial, and, yes, psychedelic applications. Each day starts with a guided forage through the alpine forests surrounding the town, followed by classes and lectures, cooking demonstrations, and some really off-the-wall parties. And if mushrooms ain't your thing, no worries, Telluride hosts a festival nearly every weekend in the summer, celebrating everything from blues music to nature films.

Seattle

While most of the post-legalization media attention has focused on Colorado, the great state of Washington also voted to free the weed, on November 6, 2012, and—after getting a slower start out of the gate—the Emerald City now boasts a marijuana scene every bit as vibrant and vital as the Mile-High City, only with a decidedly West Coast flair.

For where to stay in town, again, a growing number of Bud-and-Breakfasts openly court cannabis tourists, or you can always get together with a few friends and rent something on

VRBO or Airbnb—after confirming that the owner's cool with you getting totally blazed on the premises.

Meanwhile, if you really want to jump in lungs-first, there's no better time to visit than the third weekend in August, when the city plays host to **Seattle Hempfest,** which started in 1991 as a humble assembly of local stoners and has since grown into the world's largest annual gathering of advocates for the legalization of marijuana. Drawing more than 80,000 attendees daily for three days to Seattle's waterfront **Myrtle Edwards Park** for music, speeches, vendors, amusements, and more, Hempfest attracts the nation's leading marijuana activists, entrepreneurs, and even celebrities like Woody Harrelson. And if you're wondering how the "city fathers" feel about such a massive ganja party happening right under their noses, keep in mind that at the first Hempfest after Washington State legalized it, both major candidates for mayor addressed the crowd to make clear their unwavering support, while the Seattle Police Department handed out bags of Doritos tagged with friendly suggestions for how to enjoy legal cannabis safely and responsibly.

My other favorite stoned pastime in town is a visit to **Pike Place**, a nine-acre, hundred-year-old public market overlooking the majestic Elliott Bay. Home to farmers, butchers, fishmongers, cheesemongers, bakers, winemakers, and countless other local purveyors, plus one of the largest craft markets in the country, featuring all locally made handcrafted goods, Pike Place ranks among the finest places to take a stoned stroll in America. Rather than sit down for a single meal, I suggest trying a small snack from a wide selection of stalls, making sure to hit **Mee Sum Pastry, Beecher's Handmade Cheese, Uli's Famous Sausage**, and **Piroshky Piroshky Bakery**. In between noshes, take time to visit the anarchist-friendly **Left Bank Books**, and reportedly one of America's oldest head shops.

At night, I've wasted some fun hours in Seattle with the *High Times* crew at **Add-a-Ball**, an aggressively casual pinball bar in the city's lively Fremont neighborhood. Home to artists, bohemians, and political dissidents, and known locally as "the center of the universe," Fremont boasts countless fun places to eat, drink, and experience life, plus, under the Aurora Bridge, there's an eighteen-foot-tall concrete sculpture of a troll crushing a Volkswagen Beetle. Or, for something a bit more highbrow, check out **Chihuly Garden and Glass**, which is absolutely one of the trippiest museums on Earth (where you're also likely to run into your mom), and it's located close to the **Space Needle** and **Experience Music Project**.

For more canna-specific suggestions, check out the "High List," a marijuana events calendar maintained by Seattle's alt-weekly the *Stranger* that highlights not just pot-friendly events but also "nearby snacks." And be sure to pick up a copy of *Dope* magazine and *Northwest Leaf* when you arrive (they should have them at the first pot store you visit) for a more in-depth look at the local scene.

Washington Highlight: Orcas Island

The largest of the San Juan Islands, located off the northwest corner of Washington State, Orcas Island boasts miles of rugged coastline frequently visited by the majestic whales that give the island its name. With less than 5,000 full-time inhabitants, this remote getaway remains largely unspoiled, and can only be reached by ferry, which means getting there truly is part of the fun (just don't get caught blazing on board!).

As for where to stay, at the risk of overrunning a lovely hidden gem, those looking for a place to enjoy the state's copious legal marijuana in a stunning natural environment without breaking the bank should strongly consider the "glamping" options afforded by **Doe Bay**, a hundred-year-old rustic resort with lovely yurts, an organic garden to supply their top-notch on-site café, and a spa with soaking tubs that look out over the ocean.

Portland

I'm not saying *Portlandia* is a factually accurate depiction of life in the city that gave birth to **Casa Diablo**—the world's first vegan strip club—but I do recommend getting really, *really* baked and watching a few episodes at home before deciding whether or not Portland's your ideal stoner vacation destination. Some people find the idea of a place "where young people go to retire" a bit off-putting, after all, but personally, I've had nothing but great times in Stumptown.

No matter what time I arrive, day or night, each visit invariably begins (and likely ends) with a trip to the original **Voodoo Doughnut** shop, a twenty-four-hour bakery whose Portland Creme the mayor once honored as the city's official doughnut. And oh yeah, they also make a Maple Blazer Blunt in honor of the local basketball team that resembles a fat, cinnamon-dusted Philly Blunt cigar—plus other off-the-wall creations featuring toppings like Cap'n Crunch cereal, crushed Oreos, maple-bacon, toasted coconut, banana chunks, cinnamon, Tang, and even a tart dusting of lemonade/iced-tea crystals on the Arnold Palmer. No wonder the place is full of drooling herbal enthusiasts at both 4:20 P.M. and A.M.

Meanwhile, for decidedly more substantial meals, you really can't do any better than visiting Portland's more than five hundred "street feeders," a movable feast of food trucks and carts that typically congregate together in what locals call "pods"—more than forty of which are scattered around the city. Start by locating the pod closest to where you're currently hungry, or make a pilgrimage to the largest and most established, at **SW**

Ninth/Tenth and Alder. Either way, come hungry, and bring weed, because you'll want to hit multiple carts, and with their low prices and generous portions you just might require a little appetite stimulation between courses.

While in town, I also always try to make a pilgrimage to **Powell's City of Books,** one of America's biggest and best independent bookstores (it's so big, in fact, they provide you with a map for getting around). Once you pick up something to read, head over to the **World Famous Cannabis Cafe,** a pioneering marijuana lounge that's been open since 2002. While there, you can get high with the locals, enjoy a beverage, and thumb through a copy of *Oregon Leaf,* a monthly newspaper easily found at Portland's marijuana stores.

Also, check out **Portland Hempstalk** in September for a truly homegrown marijuana festival, or the city's official **Waterfront Blues Festival** in July for top-flight music and a great party vibe.

Oregon Highlight: Timberline

Smoke all the dabs you want in Portland, but there's just no way to get higher in Oregon than by visiting Mount Hood, whose 11,239-foot peak marks the top elevation in the state. A national forest surrounds the mountain, with world-class hiking, hot springs, and gorgeous old-growth forest, but what makes the place truly special is a skiing/snowboarding season that lasts all year, providing North America's only "endless winter."

To find this magical realm, orient toward a spot on the southwestern face of the mountain called Timberline, a decidedly herb-friendly community of ski bums that also boasts a lively skateboarding scene. And while you're there, be sure to track down a fat sack of Jager, a local Oregon *indica*-dominant strain with an extremely high potency and a wonderful licorice taste.

Alaska

Marijuana has been decriminalized in Alaska since the 1970s, but voters only fully legalized the herb in November 2014 (along with Oregon and Washington, DC). Personally, I've never been to the forty-ninth state, but I do love the idea of embarking on a "Baked Alaska" adventure. Perhaps I'll head off into the bush in search of the elusive Matanuska Thunder Fuck strain, an Alaska-bred marijuana variety that's reported to thrive in the subarctic climate of the rugged Matanuska borough (about an hour north of Anchorage). Legend has it that just a few puffs of this powerful herb per day makes the coldest, bleakest winter bearable.

In the meantime, never having been, I can't honestly offer much travel advice beyond what you can find in a guidebook, especially since, as the first "red state" to legalize it, Alaska doesn't exactly have a lot of overt marijuana culture to offer. Though it is awfully nice to know you can now enjoy some of the most remote and unspoiled wilderness left on Earth while getting totally, legally blazed.

Amsterdam

Much has changed in the Netherlands since I first traveled to Amsterdam in 2002 to work on the video crew at the *High Times* Cannabis Cup. Once the Promised Land for marijuana enthusiasts from all over the world, the city now feels a bit behind the times. Because while patrons in several US states can buy up to an ounce of lab-tested, fully legal herb in a government-licensed store, the entire weed system—from cultivation to distribution—remains half in shadows in Holland. And lately things have been heading in the wrong direction.

For starters, the Dutch never "legalized" marijuana. Since the 1970s, they've simply "tolerated" possession of small amounts (up to 5 grams) and sale of same from a recognized coffeeshop. Commercial growing and transporting have always been a "don't ask, don't tell" proposition at best, meaning that even the most aboveboard coffeeshop owners are constantly forced to break the law just to run their businesses. And now, the bitter irony is that as the rest of the world moves toward tolerance and liberty, the Netherlands has been making life increasingly difficult for cannabis suppliers and consumers—using zoning laws to close hundreds of locations in Amsterdam alone, and in more conservative parts of the country, banning foreigners from patronizing the shops.

Aside from being a total bummer, this creeping loss of freedom also represents a serious cautionary tale for America's suddenly ascendant marijuana movement, namely that the political winds blow in two directions. In the Netherlands, for example, the recent anti-cannabis political environment comes not from any significant change in societal attitudes about the herb but rather from the unrelated election of conservative, religious, anti-immigration politicians who want to repress marijuana culture along with everything else they fear and misunderstand. So next time you smoke some pot, definitely put it in the air that cooler heads will soon prevail.

In the meantime, Amsterdam remains an amazing place to visit, whether you like to get high or not. Despite all the recent closures, hundreds of coffeeshops remain open and ready to serve you throughout the city, and unlike anywhere in America (so far), you're more than welcome to not just buy herb and hash but to pull up a seat and get high. I've now been to Amsterdam at least ten times (who's counting?), and my favorite coffeeshops include two of the biggest and best known—**Green**

House and **Barney's Uptown**—though I also enjoy more intimate, quirky spots like **Mellow Yellow** (the city's first coffeeshop, since 1972), **De Dampkring**, and **Resin**.

If you want reasonably priced, extremely pot-friendly accommodations right in the heart of the city (and that ain't easy to find!), check out the **Get Lucky** guesthouse, which overlooks the Keizersgracht (King's Canal) in the stylish Rembrandtplein neighborhood (named for the Dutch master). Or better yet get a few friends together and rent a houseboat for a truly unique experience.

Although Amsterdam is better known as a place to party than a food destination, I've spent enough time in the city to have a few favorite eats. Start off any day in Amsterdam right with a visit to **Pannenkoekenhuis Upstairs** for a taste of traditional *pannenkoeken* served in an old Dutch house that dates to 1539 (OK, start the day with coffee and weed at a coffeeshop, and then get the pancakes). Also, don't miss tasting local cheese and chocolate from countless fine purveyors, or hitting up one of the various street vendors selling pickled herring, a national delicacy that arrives fresh and briny with no "fishy" taste at all. (Some places slice it into bite-size pieces and provide toothpicks, but the locals just pick them up by the tail and eat them like a cartoon cat does.)

Worthwhile marijuana tourist spots include the **Hash, Marijuana & Hemp Museum**, which isn't big but does an excellent job of representing the world's most beneficial plant, and the **Cannabis College**, which often hosts fun social occasions. Or just rent a bicycle and plot out a coffeeshop crawl on your own. (Be sure to crisscross **Vondelpark** a few times, as it's a real stunner and one of the best places in the city to puff al fresco—just make sure you find a remote spot away from the crowds.)

And as for that famous nightlife, I recommend starting the

evening at one of the city's centuries-old brown cafés, with pints of dark Dutch beer and a plate of aged Gouda cheese. From there, I love hanging out at a converted squat turned anarchist collective called **OT301**, which has a café with food and live music, a movie theater, and a dance club (check out Ping-Pong night on Tuesdays!). For hot jazz with no cover, try **Café Alto** or head to the **Melkweg** for bigger acts in an herb-friendly environment. Or just wander along the canals taking in the amazing beauty of this free-spirited, wonderfully tolerant city.

Barcelona

Barcelona's recently been dubbed "The New Amsterdam" by Europe's millions of marijuana tourists, and with good reason, since hundreds of openly operating cannabis retailers and lounges currently serve residents and foreigners, who typically sign a quick membership agreement in exchange for the right to buy and smoke cannabis on-site. Much like their counterparts in the Netherlands, the Barcelona clubs aren't officially licensed or sanctioned by any government agency but instead operate based on laws passed decades ago that permit individuals to form a cannabis club to collectively grow and consume marijuana, provided it's a nonprofit organization and all the cannabis remains within the collective.

I haven't had the good fortune to visit Spain in nearly a decade, but from everything I've read lately, and more important what I've heard firsthand from local activists, there's currently a push for more formal recognition of these "social clubs," including some level of official regulation. But for now they continue to operate in a gray area, including occasional government enforcement raids, though they've been increasingly tolerated by the police since legalization passed in the United States in 2012.

So suffice it to say, with a little advance research you'll have no problem finding high-quality cannabis and a friendly place to blaze it in Barcelona. Now, as for what to do there once you're stoned, my best times in the city involved wandering up and down the miles of beach smoking spliffs, drinking cervezas, and meeting locals, then heading inland and elbowing up to a tapas bar (somewhere away from the overly touristy La Rambla) for local Rioja wine and small plates of regional cured meats, cheeses, peppers, and olives, plus special delicacies like setas al ajillo (mushrooms in oil and garlic), patatas braves (fried potato diced in a spicy tomato sauce), boquerones en vinagre (anchovies in vinegar), and my personal favorite, bacalao (thinly sliced deep-fried cod).

Please note that *tapas* literally means "small plate," so each dish arrives as just a few perfect bites, on a serving vessel originally designed to rest on top of a wineglass, in order to keep the flies out of your vino.

Visit Barcelona in March to catch **Spannabis,** one of Europe's largest marijuana events, which draws a huge international crowd to the city annually to celebrate all things *mota*. The festival includes seminars with leading growers, activists, and entrepreneurs; booths selling everything from seeds to trimming machines; and a bunch of amazing pot parties. Also, don't miss the mind-bending architectural marvels built by **Gaudí** (all around the city), and the beautiful views from the top of **Montjuic Mountain.**

Jamaica

At or near the top of pretty much every stoner dream vacation list ever published, Jamaica combines tropical paradise with plentiful *sativa* and a famously pot-friendly culture, particularly among the island's sizeable Rastafarian population. Just don't head down there and act like everybody you meet must be a ganja-growing reggae singer. That's some ignorant shit.

But *do* go down there, especially if the Jamaican government follows through on plans to legalize marijuana on the island as a way to raise tax money, improve public safety, and attract tourism. Those reforms remain in development as this book goes to press, but needless to say this positive public policy change, if enacted, would have a transformative effect on the Caribbean nation, bringing a huge segment of the economy out of the shadows while allowing Jamaican citizens and foreign travelers alike an opportunity to enjoy some of the world's finest ganja together in peace.

Hopefully this new push toward freedom, openness, and herbal liberty will be led by the Rastas themselves, who deserve a chance to make a living by growing and providing the herb they've suffered and sacrificed so greatly for over the years, rather than getting pushed aside by powerful homegrown business interests and the international pot industry. You can do your part by pouring your tourist dollars into the island's true grassroots cannabis community in a responsible way by spending the extra time to seek out high-quality, well-run independent hotels, restaurants, and tour companies with a true local connection (rather than a corporate overlord).

Also, no ganja tour of Jamaica would be complete without a visit to the **Bob Marley Museum** in Kingston and **Nine Miles**, the legendary reggae singer-songwriter's place of birth, which also boasts a museum dedicated to his music, life, and legacy. Otherwise, as always, eschew the overrun tourist beaches and all-inclusive resorts in favor of seeking out more authentic experiences, like hiking and camping in **Blue and John Crow Mountains National Park**; exploring the gushing cascades, waterfalls, and rope swings at **Blue Hole**; or asking the locals where to find the best reggae music and DJ sound clashes.

HOW TO GET STONED AROUND THE WORLD (WHERE IT AIN'T QUITE LEGAL YET)

Learn time-tested tips and techniques for finding marijuana, and tapping into the local cannabis culture, wherever you may roam.

* If simple possession of personal amounts of marijuana is a serious crime where you're headed, strongly consider taking a vacation from weed, instead of a weed vacation. Marijuana's one of life's greatest pleasures, especially when "on the road," but other than serious medical use, it's just not worth risking your own freedom or causing problems for your hosts, new friends, or total strangers just to get high.

* In more amenable environments, start by seeking a friend, not a dealer. And that doesn't mean trying to make friends with the first person to offer you weed on the street (unless you want bad weed, or bunk weed, at a shitty price from a total stranger). Instead, put forth an effort to connect with someone in-country on a non-ganja-oriented level first, whether through existing contacts or by getting directly involved in the life of the place you're visiting. Then, once you make an open-minded friend whom you trust (and who trusts you), you can start the slow, delicate dance of scoring some black-market herb.

* Rather than flat-out asking for help scoring pot, ease into things slowly with a general discussion of the subject, bringing it up in a noncommittal way. For example, you might ask if there's a lively local reggae

scene. And if that doesn't spark a fruitful dialogue, you can just say something like (white lie), "I saw a guy today with marijuana leaves on his socks. Can you believe that?" Only proceed from there to more pointed questions if your "jay-dar" indicates that you've found a sympathetic fellow herbalist. Otherwise, laugh it off and suggest going out for beers.

* Remember, just because someone shares their personal stash with you, it doesn't mean they're a dealer, or comfortable helping you hook up with one. So don't ever put them on the spot.

* Always trust your instincts. Never let your love of weed and pot culture blind you to a shady person or a sketchy situation. And never carry more herb than you need or flash around a lot of currency or expensive personal possessions.

* If a new friend does help you make a green connection, most definitely acquire enough to share generously. Because what grows around, comes around!

A PLACE CALLED HIGH: GANJA AS DESTINATION

The best travel advice I've ever gotten came from the highly esteemed host of *Rick Steves' Europe* on PBS and *Travel with Rick Steves* on NPR, when I interviewed him for *High Times* shortly after his home state of Washington passed marijuana legalization—an effort he'd helped lead.

Steves told me he somehow made it all the way through college in the 1970s without so much as taking a puff, then decided to try pot for the first time while in Kabul, Afghanistan, during a formative postcollegiate journey along the famed Hippie Trail that led high-minded, adventurous young travelers from Lebanon to Bangkok back in those heady days.

"I didn't smoke in college because I felt like there was a lot of peer pressure, and I didn't want to succumb to it," he recalled. "But in Afghanistan, the whole world was high—you'd be riding a bus, and at the rest stop they'd all sit around and watch somebody slaughter a goat while passing around some sort of a pipe or bong. . . . Of course, where I really learned to enjoy the experience was in Nepal, in Katmandu. I'd get high and eat apple pie hot out of a medieval oven while listening to the Rolling Stones, surrounded by travelers from all over the world. And I'd just think, 'Life is good.'"

Steves eventually turned adventuring into a career, thanks to his profoundly simple philosophy of enhancing your travel experiences by striving to become a "temporary local," a concept he extends even to journeys that take place entirely within your own mind. As he once explained to a crowd of nearly 100,000 at the annual Seattle Hempfest.

I am a travel writer. And for me, "high" is a place. It's a beautiful place where my speakers sound better, where suddenly I'm a good cook, and where conversations slither around like stray cats. And so yes, once in a while, I like to go there. A lot of people do. Now there are instances when our government says we can't go someplace, but if they say we can't go there, they better have a good reason. And as far as I'm concerned, there's no good reason for our government to tell adults we can't go to that beautiful place called "high."

Amen to that.

My fondest wish in writing this book, in fact, is that you will come to regard this volume as a trusted and well-informed travel guide to High, one that fully embraces Rick Steves's concept of the temporary local. Because like any popular destination, you can certainly get taken in and hustled by the tourist traps and package deals of High (for example, microwave mac and cheese, binge-watching, Candy Crush), but whether you get stoned once a day or once a year, it's always worth digging a little deeper, and seeking out something a little more real.

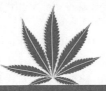

CHAPTER 7

Keep Pot Weird

*Cannabis culture must continue
stretching into the sunlight of freedom
without ever losing touch with its roots
in the underground.*

After all these years, I sometimes wonder if I'll ever get a little "burned out" on weed, not as an intoxicant, medicine, and all-around enhancement agent but as a topic of discussion. As things stand now, I'm nearing the completion of my second book on the subject, I've written extensively about the herb for nearly a third of my life, I produce a marijuana video series for VICE, and I spend a good deal of my free hours volunteering at WAMM, the world's most wonderfully compassionate medical-cannabis garden and collective. My wife also rocks a full-time pot job, and we both spend a good deal of time and energy traveling to various marijuana events, conferences, and symposiums, or heading out into the field to report on everything from an amazing new hybrid strain to a gravely unjust bust to the launch of a $75 million marijuana hedge fund.

Even when I'm out and about in a totally unrelated setting, happy to sit back and listen to some group of wholly engaging humans discuss what makes *their* worlds spin, I find that talk almost invariably swings around to my own area of expertise (especially, but not exclusively, if I happen to be getting high with said engaging humans). Not that I mind, exactly. In fact, I have a fairly evangelical feeling about *Cannabis sativa*, especially since, once we start discussing the subject in depth, I find that many of the most well-educated, open-minded, pro-cannabis people on Earth still don't know exactly *how* amazing, and potentially transformative, this species, in all forms, really is for our bodies, our minds, our spirits, and the planet we call home.

I could go on and on about that, and typically do, but then, sometimes, despite all the positive reinforcement, and the clear fact that lately the whole world has gotten a bit weed-obsessed right alongside me, I do start to think that there's surely more pressing concerns than a common green herb.

What keeps me coming back for more, then—in addition to the wonderful feeling of getting high, and the many lasting joys, allies, and epiphanies this plant has brought into my life—is the way cannabis intersects with so many other subjects I personally find fascinating. Reporting on marijuana from all angles means investigating botany, biology, chemistry, medicine, horticulture, criminal justice, technology, politics, law, economics, history, ecology, culture, and so much more—and so it never gets old. In fact, becoming a specialist in cannabis has afforded me what I consider a uniquely disillusioning education in how the world really works. And while the word "disillusioned" tends to have a negative connotation in our society, I certainly don't mean it that way. Let's just say I vastly prefer the illusion of someone pulling a rabbit out of a hat to someone pulling the wool over my eyes.

Luckily, learning the true facts about marijuana and its prohibition taught me fairly early on in life that even in the so-called information age, the powers that be can still tell big, obvious lies, with terrible consequences, and pretty much every institution of society (government, media, science, medicine, law, education, religion) will just keep dancing to the beat, as long as the piper gets paid and the band plays on.

And now legalization has come along and revealed just how quickly those same institutions all fall into line once the music stops. Consider the fact that the *Denver Post* urged every citizen in Colorado to vote against marijuana legalization in November 2012, before turning around almost immediately after it passed and launching the Cannabist, a wonderfully pro-pot website clearly designed to cash in on the attendant "green rush" of recreational weed.

Then, after decades of being treated like a laughingstock by the rest of the media, a whole slew of highbrow articles started coming out, everywhere from the *New York Times* and *Washington Post* to *Slate* and the *New Republic,* proclaiming what a forward-thinking and courageous publication *High Times* has been since starting up in 1974. Which naturally felt very flattering for a minute, until I realized they were all just covering their own asses for fucking up so royally. Because with all due respect to me and all my *High Times* colleagues—past and present—we didn't exactly puzzle together string theory. I mean, I pretty much saw through every argument against pot by the time I graduated high school, and without the aid of the Internet.

And yet the *New York Times* didn't see fit to endorse legalization until 2014, and even then the editorial board spilled far more ink patting themselves on the back for their long-overdue evolution on the issue than they did engaging in any serious examination of exactly how "the paper of record" managed to get such a simple story so wrong, for so long.

Meanwhile, despite a clear and growing national majority in

favor of sweeping reform, we still don't have a major political party in America that supports ending federal marijuana prohibition. This year, even after all our unprecedented political progress, more than 600,000 otherwise law-abiding Americans will still be arrested on marijuana charges, plus countless others around the world (with the poor and disenfranchised invariably disproportionately targeted). In most US states, cancer patients still face arrest and worse for smoking a joint to relieve the nausea of chemotherapy, even though synthetic 100 percent THC pills have been available by prescription for this exact use since 1985. Most doctors still remain wholly ignorant of the endocannabinoid system and how it could hold the key to revolutionizing modern medicine. Most religious leaders still talk about this lifesaving, nontoxic, God-given natural plant as if it were the spawn of Satan. And perhaps worst of all, far, far too many people who could really benefit from having Mary Jane in their lives still go without, out of fear of legal repercussions, social restrictions, or simply because they've internalized a century of propaganda foisted upon us by those who profit mightily off the current system and see no need to rock the boat.

When I first started following this story, by the way, all of the above was actually much, much worse (and it was even worse before that).

Fifteen years ago, publicly self-identifying as a marijuana user, or even taking it up as a political cause, pretty much disqualified you from being taken seriously in the public square. Well-meaning colleagues (almost all of them closeted pot smokers) endlessly warned me that I'd never land a "serious job" in journalism after working at *High Times* and writing about my own positive experiences with marijuana, but that honestly never really bothered me, because I couldn't then, and still can't, take seriously any person or institution that thinks they have any right to prevent me or any other adult from growing, possessing, or consuming a plant.

So I don't regret a single minute I've spent, on or off the clock, pushing back against that idea. My fondest memory of this entire journey, in fact, isn't inhaling the finest hashish in Amsterdam or joining a crew of renegade New Age ganja growers to share in the utter abundance of a NorCal outdoor pot harvest, but rather the feeling I got walking off the set of *Fox & Friends*, at Fox News headquarters in midtown Manhattan, after squaring off against some asshole from the Heritage Foundation in the wake of the great Michael Phelps bong-picture scandal of 2009.

I'd always been the kind of guy who yelled back at the television while watching those types of political debates at home, thinking how much I'd love to have my say someday, but then when my chance finally came, I seriously didn't sleep a minute the night before, as I kept gnawing over and over everything I wanted to express, and all the different ways the fine folks at Fox could conspire to make me look like an idiot in front of my own mother (and about a million other people). For a brief moment, in the darkest depths of that long night of uncertainty, I actually seriously considered just lighting up a doobie on live TV and asking what right they had to stop me. *What could they do to me, really?* But luckily, by the time dawn broke, that seemed like a pretty bad idea (for the pot movement and for me). Instead, I vowed to go on the rhetorical (rather than herbal) offensive, no matter what leading question or skewed "data" the inane hosts or my asinine opponent threw at me.

For years, I'd been watching Mason Tvert, who eventually codirected Colorado's successful marijuana legalization campaign, highlight the incredible hypocrisy of a society that enthusiastically promotes alcohol while seriously punishing those who choose cannabis, in order to make people consider the issue in a new way. From erecting billboards declaring MARI-JUANA: NO HANGOVERS. NO VIOLENCE. NO CARBS, to publicly calling brewpub pioneer turned Colorado governor John Hickenlooper a "drug dealer," Mason never misses a chance to challenge cultural norms that have us blithely cheering on a Jack Daniel's–sponsored NASCAR team while kicking down the doors of peaceful ganja smokers.

So when a cursory bit of research revealed that in 2004, long before the famous bong-toke photos hit the Internet, Michael Phelps had been arrested for a DUI, I decided to start the televised debate off by asking my opponent, point-blank, why the corporate suits at Kellogg's were apparently fine hiring an Olympic gold-medal swimmer with a drunk driving conviction on his record as a spokesperson for a sugar-coated breakfast cereal marketed to children, but then turned around and unceremoniously dropped him based on an unauthorized photo of what I can only assume, given the man's immense lung capacity, was one of the world's largest bong rips taken in a private residence.

To which Ernest James Istook Jr., former Republican member of the US House of Representatives from Oklahoma, actually replied that drinking alcohol is legal, and smoking marijuana is illegal, so that's the moral difference. Leaving me to helpfully point out that getting drunk may indeed be legal, but marijuana consumption and drunk driving are both *illegal*, even though only one of them poses any real danger—to the perpetrator and to society. Then I followed up by asking Istook how, exactly, arresting adults for consuming a natural herb with no lethal dose or serious side effects advances his organization's stated mission of promoting "free enterprise, limited government and individual freedom," because to me, marijuana prohibition actually represents an unconscionable attack on all three of those sacred principles

From there, the segment ended rather abruptly as I recall. The whole shebang lasted about two minutes, and it all went by in a dizzying flash.

What I actually best remember from that entire experience is a sort of slow-motion moment while walking off the set. I was on my way back to the woefully misnamed Fox News "green room," when I briefly caught the eye of one of the camera operators—a big, burly, bearded guy—and he gave me a very, very subtle thumbs-up. It was a simple gesture, but it's stuck with me ever since because, beyond the empathic kindness of this total stranger offering me immediate reassurance about my performance, I just loved the feeling of deep connection we shared, in the very belly of the right-wing noise machine. And looking back now, amid all the attendant excitement of marijuana moving increasingly into the mainstream, I just can't help but worry that such moments of unspoken solidarity will be fewer and further between as cannabis culture boldly enters a new post-prohibition era.

For now, serious weed heads like me, you, and that cameraman remain united by not just our shared herbal enthusiasm but also our mutual oppression. In time, when this insane War on Weed finally ends, and the world wakes up to a new green dawn, we will learn to forgive the way our kind have been abused and mistreated for championing a truly righteous cause. But we must never forget. Because to move forward otherwise, for example by making cannabis "just another consumer product like McDonald's and Budweiser," as so many well-intentioned reformers suggest, seems to me like a huge missed opportunity. I say let's not be in such a rush to fully embrace a totally fucked-up system that's still keeping us down and locking us up for no good reason. Let's not just hack away at the branches of evil, to paraphrase Henry David Thoreau, let's strike at the root.

Remember way back at the very outset of this book when I suggested that to truly secure our rights we must move beyond a "harm reduction" mind-set when it comes to marijuana, and instead start loudly and proudly celebrating the many serious benefits this plant brings into our lives and communities? Well, we've already covered marijuana's tremendous medicinal powers, the way it makes us more creative and collaborative, enhances life's pleasures, promotes meaningful social bonds, facilitates cross-cultural understanding, nurtures spirituality, and offers a far safer alternative to alcohol and many pharmaceutical drugs, but that's really just the beginning. Because as those of us who've already fully integrated cannabis into our beings know, this sorely misunderstood herb also has the potential to help us all live more meaningful, satisfying, and authentic lives while becoming more caring and compassionate friends, lovers, neighbors, parents, and citizens. And that, in turn, could transform society in a wonderfully subversive way.

Imagine waking up in a parallel universe where getting high is a widely celebrated part of life instead of a crime, a sin, a vice, or a dirty little secret. Without demonizing any other drug (or those who use them), wouldn't lots of people freely choosing pot over booze, pills, and cigarettes mean less violence, addiction, and needless suffering in the world—and a lot more peace, love, and understanding? I think so.

But we won't get there by merely making marijuana normal, because what passes for normal in our own universe is both unreasonably square and severely unjust. So those of us who know how to smoke pot properly must go beyond that. We must teach the rest of the world that it's OK to get a little weird.

LET CANNABIS HELP YOU
CULTIVATE THE WEIRD WITHIN

Marijuana is many things to many people. The herb's effects also vary widely depending on when, where, how, and why you consume it—not to mention who you consume it with. So smoking pot properly requires understanding the difference between taking massive bong hits and playing video games with your homies after a long shift at work, versus snuggling up with your significant other and a plate of fresh-baked pot cookies on a lazy Sunday. Or stopping to puff a jay on a solo hike through the forest, for that matter.

In each instance (unless you get *really* lit), it's pretty clear who you're getting high with, how you're getting high, where you're getting high, and when you're getting high, so the one question you've got to consistently ask is: *Why am I getting high?* Do you want to feel a special connection to your friends, enhance the fun of playing *Super Smash Bros.,* and break free of your workplace stress? Do you want to feel a special connection to your lover, make each other laugh, enhance sensual pleasure, and incite desire? Or do you want to feel a special connection to your own soul, embrace the untamed beauty of nature, and leave behind for a moment all distractions?

Because whether your answer to *Why am I getting high?* touches on the medicinal, the spiritual, the recreational, or a heady blend of all three, simply focusing for a moment on your intentions before lighting up will greatly increase your odds of actually realizing those intentions.

And don't worry about having a lofty goal like "achieve enlightenment" or "visualize world peace," because "make this ice cream sundae extra-delicious" also works wonders. Or better yet, how about "invent a new milkshake from what's already in the kitchen"? That intention goes beyond passive ice-cream enhancement into active creativity, and that's where weed's ability to awaken our own innate weirdness can get *really* interesting. I mean, how do you think peanut butter first met chocolate?

Anyway, to me, *getting weird* is perhaps the best of all intentions, because it's something we all so sorely lack in our day-to-day, wolf-eat-dog modern existence—a deficiency that affects our lives in many negative ways, from fostering anxiety, depression, and anger to spurring feelings of isolation and alienation. We are, after all, wild creatures taught from cradle to grave to sit up straight, face forward, and talk only when called upon. We're asked daily, even hourly, to suppress our most basic individual desires and drives in favor of the herd's demands for order and obedience. This is not a natural state of being, and so surely something's got to give.

Personally, I believe marijuana can serve as a wonderful venting mechanism for all of that pent-up weirdness to work itself out in a constructive (rather than destructive) way. Could be singing in the shower, turning a cartwheel for no reason, or deciding to plop right down in the sandbox with your five-year-old for a make-believe rocket launch. The point is to use marijuana as a way to shrug off all the pointless conventions and constraints forced upon us by society in favor of following our bliss and having fun.

Just don't ever forget the key difference between fun and entertainment.

"Everybody makes their own fun," playwright David Mamet wrote in *State and Main*. "If you don't make it yourself, it ain't fun, it's entertainment."

So while there's certainly nothing wrong (and a lot right!) with occasionally rolling up a fatty and binge-watching some Netflix, if that ever becomes your default way to unwind, then it's time to get less entertained and start having more fun, because you're not getting the most out of the herb, or your life. In such an instance, I'd suggest going right on smoking weed while simultaneously ridding yourself of the dangerous, addictive narcotic known as television (or video games, or social media, or whatever else has been pulling you down into a rut). Then get into something a bit more engaging instead—a process that begins, as always, with deciding what you will do after you get high, *before* you get high.

To help you get started, here's a few suggestions for stoned endeavors that cater to, and help cultivate, the weird within. . . .

KEEP A JOURNAL: Sitting quietly and scribbling your stoned thoughts onto an otherwise blank page might not look "weird" from the outside, but you'll quickly discover that taking the time to express your innermost feelings without an outside audience will take you to some strange and illuminating places.

PLAY CHARADES: I would actually prefer to advise you to "play make-believe," but most adults, no matter how faded, tend to cringe a bit at that particular phrasing. Still, the imperative to pretend to be something other than our "normal" selves is a basic human desire, one we should all wholeheartedly embrace from time to time. And getting blazed first can really help you get over yourself, and get into character.

MAKE SOMETHING: Marijuana only boosts creativity if you actually create. So paint a picture, write a song, build a snowman, design a bookcase . . . it really doesn't matter what you make, as long as you find the process enjoyable. And be sure to take on a project from time to time with absolutely no practical use beyond its own existence, as that precise lack of utilitarian purpose is actually your cultural license to get as weird as you'd like.

PUSH YOUR BOUNDARIES: Make a conscious decision to get high and then do something you've never done before, or go somewhere you've never gone before, which could mean anything from trying out a new sport to sampling a new kind of food to spending a night at the opera. You may end up finding disc golf dull, Cambodian cuisine unpalatable, and that *La Bohème* lasts about two hours too long, but even then, you'll be better off for having tried. And on the flip side, you just might find a new favorite pastime.

DANCE: We humans have been moving our bodies to the beat for roughly as long as we've been getting baked, so if you already like to dance, getting high and dancing will likely come quite naturally. But for the rest of us, who may feel shy or inhibited when it comes to cutting a rug, I can only say that you've got to at least try this combination, even if you can only "dance like nobody's watching" when literally nobody's watching.

BE A FLANEUR: Leave it to the French to have a long-running appreciation of the art of wandering around without a set agenda or destination. Initially the word *flâneur* had a decidedly negative connotation associated with laziness or lack of purpose, but then in the nineteenth century, intellectuals associated with Paris's Club des Hashischins, including Baudelaire and Balzac, recast the idea in a positive light, no doubt after taking the long, weird way home from a cannabis-and-coffee-soaked meeting of their famed hashish club.

NEVER STOP HANGING
HEAVY WITH YOUR BEST BUDS

There's nothing wrong with being a loner stoner if that's your thing. As a writer, I certainly fit the bill more often than not as I actively pursue my vocation, and even when I'm not working, the pleasures of a good book and a fat joint enjoyed in total seclusion are far from lost on me.

But I also find that to truly smoke pot properly, it's essential to get high with some fellow humanoids on the regular too—for the fun of it, of course, and also to balance out a kind of techno-isolation bubble that seems to come along with existence these days. Just remember, when blazing with a friend, same thing goes as always, only double. And that's decide what you will do after you get high, before you get high, and then do it.

Also, try to place equal importance on keeping truly connected to your OG smoking circle, and continually branching out and meeting new and interesting people who share your love of weed. Remember the old saying: Make new friends and keep the old, one is Super Silver Haze and the other is Acapulco Gold.

PRO TIP

EMBRACE DIVERSITY

"When I think of the people I have smoked pot with, they're such an eclectic mix of people, and I probably never would have spoken to a lot of them if it weren't for pot."

—DAVE CHAPPELLE, *HIGH TIMES*

BE A TOKIN' WOMAN

Throughout this last century of global cannabis prohibition, the cultivation and distribution of marijuana—like most other criminal enterprises—has been overwhelmingly male-dominated. But it wasn't always this way. In fact, going all the way back to prehistory and the earliest foraging societies, women typically took the lead as both herb gatherers and plant medicine healers.

So what happened?

For starters, as we moved from small, polytheist, matriarchal societies to large, monotheist, patriarchal societies, pretty much everything on Earth became less grassroots and more hierarchical, allowing men to seize control of the means of cannabis production, distribution, and so much more. Female healers also became a frequent target of witch-hunts and other coordinated campaigns of eradication, as they represented a serious threat to both "religion" and "medicine," at least as practiced by male priests and male doctors. So that by the time our modern War on Weed rolled around about a hundred years ago, the very idea of sacred plant medicine was considered "quackery" by most Americans, while single pharmaceutical compounds derived from those very same plants were hailed as "miracle drugs."

The good news is that marijuana's increasing cultural and legal acceptance has begun to close the ganja gender gap at last. And while the media only got excited once they discovered "stiletto stoners"—or "smart, successful" women with "killer careers" and "enviable social lives," according to the *Marie Claire* article that officially spotted the trend—the marijuana movement has actually long benefited from the amazing courage and conviction of our culture's true OG females, who come from all walks of life, and serve the herb as growers, dealers, healers, artists, activists, entrepreneurs, and political leaders.

They also proudly represent a tradition that goes back to antiquity, according to Ellen Komp, a longtime cannabis activist and deputy director of California NORML, whose blog *Tokin Woman* (tokinwoman.blogspot.com) has celebrated "famous female cannabis connoisseurs" since 2008.

"When I give presentations about cannabis's 'herstory' to women, including stories about the Sumerian goddess Ishtar, the Egyptian goddess Seshat, the Hindu goddess Parvati, and the Chinese goddess Magu—they come up to me afterwards and say, 'You've made me feel like I'm a part of something,'" Ellen told me recently, explaining that she's soon to publish a book on the subject, because "now is the time to heal humanity, and the planet, with the return of our plant allies and the women who respect and represent them."

Amen to that. Also, never forget that it's the female cannabis plant we all revere for getting us high and relieving our ailments.

IN PRAISE OF CANNABIS COUPLES

Couples that blaze together stay together, due to marijuana's unparalleled ability to increase intimacy, foster communication, and promote empathy. At least, that's been my experience, and I know my wife agrees. Cannabis also fuels some of our most fun, and fruitful, brainstorming sessions, and enhances many other activities we both enjoy, like cooking a meal together, walking the dogs, and gardening. Plus, having weed in the house means we can sort of take a pleasing little thirty-minute vacation anytime we want. And smoking the peace pipe really works wonders for conflict resolution.

Now, as far as I know, there's never been a serious scientific study of romantic couples where both partners use marijuana to see if they have more honest, egalitarian, supportive, engaging, amusing, mutually empowering relationships, but I've certainly seen a lot of anecdotal evidence suggesting this might be the case. In fact, I've encountered literally hundreds of bonded pairs who share a passion for cannabis at various marijuana events and in the course of my reporting, and they all just seem a little more attuned to each other than the average couple.

I certainly had that feeling right away the first time I talked with Ben Sinclair and Katja Blichfeld, a dedicated cannabis couple and cocreators of the critically acclaimed HBO series *High Maintenance,* which follows the adventures of an unnamed pot-delivery guy as he pedals his way through New York City. Married on New Year's Eve 2010, they began writing the first episode six months later (it premiered as an independent web series in 2013), and have since enjoyed a slow, steady climb from cult hit to critical darling to huge ads on the sides of public buses and tall buildings in Brooklyn, where most of the protagonist's deals go down.

I really, really love the show, and I especially love the way Sinclair and Blichfeld portray marijuana users—our diversity and complexity—without falling back on any tired stereotypes. So how exactly do they incorporate the herb into their own lives and their complicated relationship while wearing so many hats at once? And what advice can they offer to all the other cannabis couples in the world?

"We personally are both regular marijuana users, and the way we portray it on the show is pretty much reflective of our feelings," Blichfeld told me for a VICE feature. "That includes times where we feel like maybe we're smoking too much, and not just for financial reasons. Perhaps we're smoking to avoid dealing with personal issues, or some adult responsibilities that we're not looking forward to having to face. But ultimately we use it as medicine, to relieve stress, and to enhance our creativity.

Weed definitely helps to calm the anxious voice in my head when Ben and I are gearing up to do some writing. We like to smoke and then go for a walk to brainstorm. It's not that we can't be creative without the aid of marijuana, but it really has facilitated the birth of so many of our best ideas! It kind of opens our minds up to possibilities. Also, we're emotional people and pot helps us bounce back from conflicts quickly. I'm prone to getting flooded with emotion, while Ben is prone to anger. The weed soothes us both and helps us empathize with each other."

"Pot gets ahead of the anger before it blinds you," Sinclair added, "and allows you to come back to a more watercolor version of the world, where the lines aren't so drawn in the sand. They're more muddled, relaxed, and impressionistic and it doesn't feel so hot in the room. Also, when I'm editing, I smoke—a lot—because I'm stuck there at my computer for days on end, and weed helps me get into a flow zone where that time just disappears, and I can just let it go. Getting started can be tough when you're stoned, but once you're there, it's really fun to move clips around and explore the possibilities. I stop judging myself so much and start to just play. Which also works in a relationship."

REEFER DADNESS (AND MOMNESS TOO)

The sad fact is that we live in a world where parents who consume cannabis instead of drinking alcohol (or popping Xanax or disappearing into the tube or the net) face being stigmatized by their friends and family, not to mention potentially suffering far worse sanctions from their employers, law enforcement, and Child Protective Services—even for responsible marijuana use, and even in states where the herb's been fully legalized. So any parent or guardian with minors in the house needs to make extremely clearheaded decisions when it comes to getting high.

Store all cannabis and paraphernalia out of sight, in clearly labeled containers, in a locking box, along with a copy of your doctor's recommendation if you have one. Never discuss marijuana with, or get high in front of, someone who could use that information against you. Never do anything that would put yourself or your children in jeopardy. And make a plan for the worst-case scenario, including knowing the attorney you will contact in case of emergency.

Also, don't ever let society make your feel guilty or inferior for choosing cannabis. Because when you consider everything we objectively know about marijuana's safety and its effects on consciousness, plus the fact that (perfectly legal and widely accepted) alcohol is a leading cause of spousal and child abuse, it seems exceedingly clear that allowing parents to access the herbal option without worry would in most cases make for far more attentive, intuitive, peaceful caregivers.

Until very recently, however, few would make that argument in public, as even marijuana's staunchest supporters tended to shy away from talking about children and parenting whenever possible, rather than risk alienating middle-of-the-road folks who can accept that simple possession of marijuana shouldn't send you to jail, but still think "parenting while high" should be a felony. (Again, only provided you're high on pot and not Pinot Noir or pain pills).

A wonderful 2012 *Jezebel* post titled "I'm a Mom and I'm Stoned Right Now," for example, was published anonymously, lest it incite a real-life (rather than online) clash between the herbally inclined author and a bunch of naysayers. In the funny, insightful essay, "Stoned Mom" opened by admitting:

I wanted to get my husband to watch our daughter so I could get stoned and pound out this essay about being a mom who smokes pot. But when I stepped back into our apartment after smoking about half a bowl of something called "purple train wreck" out on the terrace, I knew I'd never be able to get any work done with this cute ass baby around to distract me. In the middle of playing some totally vacant, rule-less game that involved pretending to chew stuff, making growling noises, and giggling, I realized that she's like the funniest fucking person I've ever met. Anybody who thinks that weed makes parents ignore their children has clearly never been high around one.

The essay must have struck a chord, because within two months, an only slightly tongue-in-cheek *New York Times* opinion piece by Mark Wolfe made basically the same argument, from the Reefer Dadness point of view:

After two years of [medical-marijuana] treatment, I can state unequivocally that . . . the best part is an amazing off-label benefit I call Parental Attention Surplus Syndrome.

Before beginning treatment, I was a dutiful if not particularly enthusiastic father. Workaday parental obligations were a necessary, unfortunate chore. I was so stressed out by the end of the day that bedtime, with its interminable pleas for more stories, songs, sips of water and potty breaks, felt like a labor to be endured and dispatched as quickly as possible. . . . [But] I swear I am a more loving, attentive and patient father when I take my medication as prescribed. Perhaps this isn't surprising. As anyone who inhaled during college can attest, cannabis enhances the ability to perceive beauty, complexity and novelty in otherwise mundane things (grout patterns in your bathroom floor, the Grateful Dead, Doritos), while simultaneously locking you into a prolonged state of rapt attention. . . . [And] I submit

*that this can be enormously salutary to the parent-toddler
relationship. Beyond food, shelter and clothing, what do small
children need most from their parents? Sustained, loving, par-
ticipatory attention. Thank you, Doctor.*

So definitely don't feel like you're the only parent out there
waiting twenty minutes after putting the kids to bed, to be sure
they're really sleeping, before sneaking up to the attic for a
quick appointment with Dr. Bong. Or who believes that a puff
or two enhances everything from finger painting and mud pies
to playing hide-and-seek or chowing down on a fried bologna
sandwich.

In fact, you should feel good about showing your kids that
freewheeling, fun-loving, weird side of yourself from time to
time. Children need to see adults having fun or they won't want
to grow up!

SUPER SILVER HAZE

Long before California legalized medical cannabis in 1996, a
little old lady named Mary Jane Rathbun—but far better known
to her many admirers as Brownie Mary—took the law into her
own hands. Once named Volunteer of the Year by the AIDS
ward of San Francisco General Hospital, she baked more than
1,500 brownies per month at the height of her operation, all of
them infused with marijuana trim and shake supplied by phil-
anthropic local dealers and growers.

Eventually, her tiny apartment couldn't contain the smell of
all that baking, an aromatic overflow that led to her first of several arrests.

The authorities repeatedly threatened to throw the book at

Brownie Mary, but instead of backing down, she called bullshit, arriving for court adorned in pot-leaf jewelry and pro-legalization buttons, and basically daring her prosecutors to convince a San Francisco jury to convict a bleeding-heart granny for giving away pot brownies to AIDs patients. Only twice were they successful, and each time she was sentenced only to community service — or basically no punishment at all for a woman who selflessly worked to help others until she died in 1999, at age seventy-seven.

Today, her legend and legacy continue to inspire those who see cannabis as a social-justice issue of the highest order, but unfortunately, when it comes to actually making marijuana legalization a political reality, Mary Jane Rathbun's generation remains by far the most strongly opposed voting bloc. In 2012, for example, Colorado managed to pass legalization handily, even though exit polls showed that senior citizens opposed the measure by a 2–1 margin.

Lately, however, those numbers have begun to shift in a more positive direction, as our elders increasingly discover that marijuana provides profound, all-natural therapeutic benefits for those suffering with a variety of common geriatric conditions — from arthritis, chronic pain, and insomnia to Alzheimer's and even depression.

"When we started a couple of years ago, seniors didn't talk about marijuana, and the media definitely didn't talk about seniors and marijuana, but that's all changed," activist Robert "Black Tuna" Platshorn explained to me for a VICE story on his Silver Tour, which works to educate the country's most consistent voting bloc about the many proven benefits of medical cannabis.

I'd actually first interviewed Platshorn nearly ten years earlier, a call that kept getting interrupted by a recorded voice on the line reminding me that I was talking with a federal inmate.

In fact, prior to his release, Platshorn spent more time behind bars for marijuana than any other American ever has, and likely ever will, serving nearly three decades in federal prison on a first-time, nonviolent smuggling conviction.

And why so harsh a sentence back in an era when similar charges typically netted a suspended sentence? Turns out the case against Platshorn represented the first joint effort of the DEA and the FBI to investigate profits from the marijuana trade, and the newly empowered "Drug Warriors" decided to make an example out of him. The case therefore served as a sneak preview of many shady tactics the government would hone and expand over the next few decades, including sweeping surveillance, sleazy paid informants, so-called expert witnesses, selective prosecution, inflated statistics, overt propaganda, naked self-promotion, and, most of all, a policy of heartless ass-covering that would make War on Drugs founder Richard Nixon proud.

Set free at last in 2008, Platshorn self-published the memoir he'd started writing in prison, hoping to sell the film rights and spend his golden years sport fishing in the Florida Keys. But then, while onstage at the 2010 Seattle Hempfest, in the middle of telling an old smuggling tale that had the crowd at the nation's largest pro-pot event spellbound, he suddenly realized that preaching to the choir felt great, but accomplished little. Meanwhile, nobody seemed to be reaching out to people his age with a message tailored to their unique needs and concerns. So Platshorn started organizing informational seminars at retirement communities near his South Florida home, where the promise of a free buffet guaranteed him a captive audience willing to listen to just about anything with an open mind. Next, he raised more than $10,000 on Kickstarter to produce a twenty-eight-minute video called *Should Grandma Smoke Pot?*, and began airing it as an infomercial.

Since then he's led large groups of seniors to lobby their government in Washington, DC, and at various state capitals, and he's earned positive press coverage for the Silver Tour in the *Wall Street Journal* and the *New York Times* (plus feature segments on CNN and *The Daily Show*). And most important, he's convinced an untold number of seniors to not only support medical marijuana as a political cause but to try it themselves. So how does he suggest talking to the old folks in your life about weed?

- **EXPLAIN THE TRUE HISTORY OF MARIJUANA AND HOW IT WAS OUTLAWED:** In order to unlearn all the lies and deceptions they've been taught about this plant and those who consume it, seniors must know the real truth about the institutional racism and political opportunism that made this awful prohibition possible.

- **START THE DISCUSSION WITH HOW SAFE MARIJUANA IS:** Platshorn says seniors "want to know that there's no such thing as a fatal overdose, that it's not toxic or habit forming, that marijuana won't interfere or interact with the medications they're already taking, and that there are ways to use this medicine without smoking."

- **CITE SOURCES THEY TRUST:** Don't expect someone of any age who's opposed to, or even just afraid of, marijuana to change their mind simply because you say so. Instead, find out what conditions they have that cannabis can help relieve, and then make sure you find a source they respect to make the case. And keep in mind, older folks will likely put a lot more faith in an article published in the *New England Journal of Med-*

icine, or even just *Popular Science*, than a "mind-blowing" Joe Rogan podcast.

* **MAKE IT PERSONAL:** After you've allayed their fears
  about marijuana's safety, and cited experts to back
  yourself up, it's time to tell the old folks a story about
  someone their own age who's seen great benefit from
  using marijuana. Ideally, this would be a friend or relative you both know, but if not, I would certainly suggest mentioning that Willie Nelson is now an
  octogenarian and he still finds the energy to play hundreds of sold-out concerts all over the country every
  year.

NOTES FROM THE UNDERGROUND

*Final thoughts on marijuana as a symbol of solidarity, resistance
and freedom.*

For the most part, I strongly agree with the late, great
Groucho Marx, who famously said he'd never want to join any
club that would have someone like him for a member. Which
means I don't tend to take things like nationalism, religion,
where I went to school, my employer, my favorite band, or my
local sports team to heart. But marijuana's different, for reasons
I trust I've made clear by now.

I'm proud to be a part of cannabis culture, and I do feel a
special connection to those who share my deep reverence for
this plant. I also recognize our shared struggle, which didn't end
when the first US state legalized but will go on until all are free,
including those currently locked up as part of this unconscio-

nable botanical vendetta. As Eugene V. Debs put it in his famous
federal court statement in 1918:

> While there is a lower class I am in it, while there is a criminal
> element I am of it; while there is a soul in prison, I am not free.

And so, in closing, I'd like to suggest that smoking pot properly requires fully exercising and enjoying the liberties we've
already won, and robustly utilizing all the highs that come with
it while also remaining steadfastly radical and uncompromising
in our efforts to extend these same inalienable rights to every
herbalist on Earth. That alone will not "solve all the world's
problems," but it certainly seems to me like a great place to
start. So together, let's free the weed, and the rest will follow.

We're not there yet, but I do see a lighter at the end of the
tunnel.

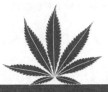

ACKNOWLEDGMENTS

The author wishes to acknowledge the start-to-finish excellent work of Kate Napolitano, who expertly shepherded this effort from its earliest conception to its final edit with her wise counsel, sustained encouragement, and indispensable eye for detail.

Alex Glass, of Glass Literary Management, has had my back for more than a decade, and I wouldn't have it any other way.

Many thanks to all my colleagues at *High Times*, past and present, for loving cannabis before it was cool, fighting the man, and having a damn good time doing it. And to my colleagues at VICE, *Munchies*, and *Motherboard* for giving me a chance to write marijuana history in real time for the last three years (and I hope many more).

Samantha Russo for bringing this book to life with her deftly drawn, spot-on illustrations.

And the rest of the wonderful team at Plume: David Rosenthal, Aileen Boyle, Milena Brown, Alice Dalrymple, and Sabrina Bowers.

My deepest appreciation and respect to all those I've profiled, quoted, or referenced in this book: Valerie Corral, Damian Marley, Martin Lee, Danny Danko, Dr. Dustin Sulak, The Nose, Doug Fine, Weeditopia. Grow It in the Sun, DJ Short, Maureen

Dowd, Tamar Wise, Zendo Project, Scott Van Rixel, Abdullah Saeed (aka T. Kid), Anita Thompson, Keith Stroup, Chris Lantner, Aurora Leveroni, Dr. Jeffrey Hergenrather, Dr. Sanjay Gupta, Chef Gabriel Reeves, Al Aronowitz, Larry "Ratso" Sloman, Lizzie Post, Doug Benson, Susie Bright, Alex Lifeson, the Trailer Park Boys, Mike Clattenburg, Brendan Kennedy, Ras Iyah V, Kris Krane, Troy Dayton, Steve DeAngelo, Richard Lee, Andy and Pete Williams, Nathan Vardi, the Fabulous Furry Freak Brothers, Captain Zero, Freddie Gibbs, Kayvan Khalatbari, Rick Steves, Mason Tvert, Ellen Komp, Ben Sinclair and Katja Blichfeld, and Robert Platshorn.

And to anyone, anywhere, who's ever stood up for the herb.

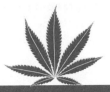

INDEX

Note: Page numbers in *italics* indicate recipes.